Breastfeeding:
A PROBLEM-SOLVING MANUAL

by

Julie M. Carroll, Dr PH
Vice President, BCA, Inc.
Public Health Nutrition Consultant

Stephen E. Saunders, MD, MPH
Chief
Division of Family Health
Illinois Department of Public Health

Carol E. Johnson, RN, PNP
Pediatric Nurse Practitioner

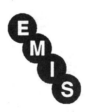

Essential Medical Information Systems, Inc.
P.O. Box 1607
Durant, OK 74702
1-800-225-0694

Direct Mail Orders
Essential Medical Information Systems, Inc.
P.O. Box 1607
Durant, OK 74702-1607

— Telephone Orders —
1-800-225-0694

— FAX Your Order —
(405) 924-9414

First Edition 1987
Second Edition 1988
Third Edition 1991
Fourth Edition 1995

ISBN: 0-929240-68-5

Printed in the United States of America

Illustrations
by:

C.W. Hoffman
Visual Communications
San Francisco

— TABLE OF CONTENTS —

— FIGURES —

— TABLES —

#1 Introduction

BREASTFEEDING PROMOTION

The Decision to Breastfeed

Breastfeeding is the mode of infant feeding recommended by the American Academy of Pediatrics, the American Public Health Association and the American Dietetic Association. In 1993, 60 percent of women giving birth in the United States initiated breastfeeding. In *Healthy People 2000, National Health Promotion and Disease Prevention Objectives,* the Surgeon General set an objective to "increase to at least 75 percent the proportion of mothers who breastfeed their babies in the early postpartum period and to at least 50 percent the proportion who continue breastfeeding until their babies are 5 to 6 months old." Breastfeeding promotion and support is essential to achieving this objective.

Promotion of breastfeeding activities should be directed towards:

- Professional groups
- The community
- Women considering and/or attempting to breastfeed

Health care providers must initiate activities that promote and support breastfeeding:

- Preconceptually
- Prenatally
- Perinatally
- Throughout the early postpartum period
- Upon mother's return to work or school

In addition, hospitals must implement policies that facilitate breastfeeding. Individuals trained as lactation consultants are becoming an important part of the health care team. They serve as resources for breastfeeding mothers, physicians and other clinicians seeing breastfeeding mothers and their babies.

Preconceptual Promotion

Studies have concluded that the majority of women make infant feeding decisions before they become pregnant. Included in this decision are such factors as:

- The woman's perception of the value and role of breastfeeding
- Influence of friends, relatives and the infant's father
- The mother's anxieties about her ability to produce sufficient high-quality milk
- The mother's future work intentions

Information on infant feeding should be included in educational programs in high school and college to provide young women and men with the basis for sound decision-making when planning to become parents.

Prenatal Promotion

Prenatally, family and friends may still influence the breastfeeding decision. However, health care providers can play a significant role in encouraging women to initiate breastfeeding. Studies indicate that patients whose health care providers actively encourage it are more likely to initiate breastfeeding. Prenatal care should include an assessment of the woman's physical ability to nurse and individualized education and counseling regarding the benefits and techniques of breastfeeding.

Participation in childbirth classes in which breastfeeding information is provided is particularly important in encouraging initiation and extended duration of breastfeeding. The level of knowledge concerning infant feeding is closely linked to the choice to breastfeed, as is the primary influence of another woman and the choice to breastfeed. Preconceptional counseling and education are particularly important for women of lower educational levels, who are less likely to initiate breastfeeding.

It is important that women considering breastfeeding be given a realistic view of it and have an understanding of the demands nursing will place on them. Education and encouragement of women to initiate breastfeeding should emphasize:

- Proper positioning of the infant for nursing (see Section #10)
- Putting the infant to the breast as soon as possible after birth, whether or not the infant successfully latches on
- An understanding of how to assess the adequacy of milk intake, i.e., six to eight wet diapers a day, stooling, adequate weight gain, etc. (see Section #16)
- That she needs to make some arrangements as soon as possible prenatally to integrate breastfeeding into her life successfully, i.e., involvement of the father or other individuals in supporting her breastfeeding
- That being flexible will make it easier to meet her own needs and the needs of the infant

8

Inclusion of the father in prenatal counseling is also desirable since, for many women, disapproval of breastfeeding by the husband or partner is enough to discourage breastfeeding. The father should be knowledgeable of:

- The benefits of breastfeeding for his mate and child
- His role and importance in the success of the breastfeeding experience through providing encouragement and support to the mother
- The mechanics of breastfeeding, i.e., positioning of the infant, manual expression of breast milk and the initial need for frequent nursing
- The importance of delaying use of rubber nipples (pacifiers and bottles) and supplemental feedings throughout the early postpartum period

Perinatal Promotion and Hospital Policies

The hospital experience strongly influences both the initiation and duration of breastfeeding. The hospital staff should be trained and available to assist breastfeeding mothers with problems that commonly arise.

Hospital policies and non-verbal teaching may be as important as the attitude and counseling provided by the staff. A number of hospitals still have policies which are relatively inflexible and do not always accurately reflect research-based information. Obstacles to successful breastfeeding include:

- Lack of early mother/infant contact and opportunity to nurse
- Hospital staff's offering supplemental water, formula or pacifiers to the breastfed infant

- Inadequately trained hospital staff
- Restricting maternal access to the baby
- Restricting feedings to every four hours
- Lack of support for overcoming common breastfeeding problems

The Baby Friendly Hospital Initiative, sponsored by the World Health Organization and United Nations International Children's Emergency Fund (1991, WHO/UNICEF), is based on 10 recommendations for hospitals. These "Ten Steps To Successful Breastfeeding" support the opportunity for successful lactation for all women. They state that hospitals should:

- Have a written breastfeeding policy that is routinely communicated to all health care staff
- Train all health care staff in the skills necessary to implement this policy
- Inform all pregnant women about the benefits and management of breastfeeding
- Help mothers initiate breastfeeding within a half hour of birth
- Show mothers how to breastfeed and how to maintain lactation even if they are separated from their infants
- Give newborn infants no food or drink other than breast milk unless medically indicated
- Practice rooming-in. Allow mothers and infants to stay together 24 hours a day
- Encourage breastfeeding on demand
- Give no artificial teats or pacifier (e.g., dummies, soothers) to breastfeeding infants
- Foster the establishment of breastfeeding support groups and refer mothers to them on discharge from hospital or clinic

Additionally, the following hospital policies will facilitate a successful breastfeeding experience:

- Minimal use of maternal medication during labor and delivery
- No separation of mother and infant post-delivery
- Allow prolonged mother/infant contact (suckling) during the first hour after delivery
- Routine distribution of breastfeeding literature and other learning aids tailored to the needs of mothers
- Elimination of elaborate nipple-washing or "duration of nursing" rituals
- No routine test weighings of full term infants to determine quantity of breast milk consumption
- No use of nipple shields
- No standing orders for anti-lactation drugs
- Discharge packs of formula given to breastfeeding mothers only upon family or physician's request

Postpartum Promotion

Most mothers are discharged from the hospital prior to the establishment of lactation. These women may experience difficulties which lead them to discontinue breastfeeding unless they receive counseling and support. The most critical period for support is within the first two weeks, and a significant number of women have expressed a desire for breastfeeding assistance during this time. In addition to counseling and support given the primary care provider, various approaches are effective in increasing the duration of breastfeeding, including:

- Postpartum telephone calls
- Peer support groups
- Breastfeeding counseling
- Follow-up
- Group classes

In addition to avoidance of early formula supplementation, the most significant factors that influence breastfeeding duration are early maternal/infant contact and support with consistent telephone follow-up. On discharge from the hospital, patients should be given specific referral, including names and telephone numbers of community resources that offer breastfeeding help, e.g., La Leche League, Special Supplemental Nutrition Program for Women, Infants and Children (WIC) or a local lactation consultant.

Mother's Return to Work or School

While returning to work or school presents a challenge to continuing breastfeeding, many women have successfully combined working and nursing. Because the return to work or school is often six or more weeks postpartum, women may no longer have ready access to health care providers. There is specific information that may be helpful to women considering returning to school or work full- or part-time.

It is not unusual for women to find the challenge of working and nursing overwhelming. It is at this time that many women discontinue nursing. Many work environments are not conducive to pumping breast milk, which requires time and a place and is necessary to continue nursing. Specific guidance for the working woman is provided in Section #4.

Demographics of Breastfeeding Mothers

In 1900, virtually 100 percent of U.S. mothers breastfed their infants. Since that time, the proportion of mothers who initiate breastfeeding has consistently declined, reaching its lowest level in 1970. From 1971 through 1982 the proportion of women initiating breastfeeding more than doubled from 25 percent to 62 percent, but between 1984 and 1989, there was a 13 percent decline in the initiation of breastfeeding and a 24 percent decline in its duration. There are regional differences in breastfeeding initiation, with the lowest rates in the South and Northeast and the highest rates in the West.

The abandonment of breastfeeding in the first half of the century began with women from the upper socio-economic level. Similarly, the resurgence of interest in breastfeeding during the last 25 years began in women of upper socio-economic status and is progressing along class lines. Women who are younger, white, affluent and college-educated are the most likely to initiate breastfeeding. In 1988, 25 percent of Black women and 51 percent of Hispanic women initiated breastfeeding, as compared to 54 percent of white women.

A large proportion of mothers terminate breastfeeding early. Approximately 25 percent are reported to discontinue breastfeeding within four weeks and 50 to 60 percent within 16 weeks postpartum.

Reasons for Discontinuation

The most common reasons for early discontinuation of breastfeeding include:

- The mother's perception of inadequate milk
- Breast engorgement
- Sore nipples
- Lack of support from health care providers

As with initiation of breastfeeding, studies indicate that poor, less-educated, young, minority mothers are more likely to discontinue breastfeeding early.

By contrast, the more enjoyable a woman finds breastfeeding and the less embarrassment she feels about nursing in public, the longer she will breastfeed.

Summary

Both the incidence and duration of breastfeeding increased from the early 1970s until the mid-1980s. Between 1984 and 1989 both decreased. As of 1993, 60 percent of women are initiating breastfeeding. Resumption of increases in the proportion of women who initiate and continue breastfeeding will require that health care providers give information and support to all women. Special emphasis must also be directed toward groups who currently are the least likely to initiate or continue breastfeeding. Adolescents, poor and minority women must receive intensive support if the goal of increasing the percentage of women who breastfeed is to be reached.

The intent of this book is to provide information that will aid health care professionals in supporting and counseling breastfeeding women effectively so that they may avoid early discontinuation of breastfeeding and have a successful experience. Preventive strategies to avoid complications of breastfeeding as well as management techniques for common problems are included in the book.

BENEFITS OF BREASTFEEDING

Breast Milk Recommended

Breast milk is the standard for infant feeding. Artificial formulas are patterned after breast milk. Breastfeeding is currently the mode of infant feeding recommended by the American Academy of Pediatrics, the American Dietetic Association and the American Public Health Association.

Breastfeeding has been demonstrated to have benefits for the infant and mother that are:
- Anti-infective
- Anti-carcinogenic
- Anti-diabetic
- Nutritional
- Anti-allergenic
- Psychological
- Convenience
- Economic
- Birth spacing

Anti-Infective Benefits

The health benefits associated with breastfeeding have been well-documented in disadvantaged populations having less than optimal sanitation, nutrition and medical care. Documenting the anti-infective benefits in more affluent populations has been more difficult due to various confounding factors, though, a lower prevalence of bacterial gastroenteritis has been clearly demonstrated. It has also been shown that infants who are exclusively breastfed have significant protection against rotavirus diarrhea; infants who are breastfed have milder symptoms of shorter duration.

Recent studies show that infants exclusively breastfed or breastfed for a longer duration are afforded some protection from acute and recurrent otitis media. This benefit to breastfed infants exists independent of cigarette smoking, group child care, allergies, numbers of siblings, gender, socio-economic status and infant's position at feeding.

Some investigators have recently examined the relationship between severe urinary tract infections and breastfeeding. While there are some indications of a protective benefit, this has not been conclusively demonstrated.

Some studies have demonstrated a reduction in respiratory illness, especially in underdeveloped countries; however, most authorities believe that any difference in reported incidence of respiratory disease is accounted for by:

- Socioeconomic status
- Parental smoking
- Day care center attendance
- Exposure to siblings

Breastfed infants appear to have lower rates of hospitalization when rates for all illnesses are combined.

Human milk contains numerous anti-infectious components not found in formula. These include:

- Immunoglobulins
- Macrophages
- Polymorphonuclear leukocytes
- T and B lymphocytes
- Bifidus factor

- Antistaphylococcal factor
- Complement lactoferrin
- Interferon

In addition to the anti-infective properties of human milk, the probability of its contamination is less than in the preparation of formulas. This protective effect is more evident in circumstances in which environmental contamination is likely, for example, where there is poor home hygiene or in developing countries. Under such situations, the mortality rate for bottle-fed infants is significantly higher than that for breastfed infants.

Anti-Carcinogenic Benefits

There is consistent evidence that women who breastfeed are at a lower risk for breast cancer. Longer duration of breastfeeding may offer even greater protection.

Infants who are breastfed longer than six months, when compared with those who are breastfed less than six months or are formula-fed, have been shown to have a lower risk of certain types of cancer.

Anti-Diabetic Benefits

Infants exposed to cow's milk early in life are at increased risk of developing insulin-dependent diabetes mellitus, as compared to infants who are exclusively breastfed. The risk increases with shorter duration of breastfeeding or earlier exposure to cow's milk. Further, diabetic children have been shown to have antibodies to cow's milk protein. Several theories about these important findings and their ramifications are currently under investigation.

Anti-Allergenic Benefits

A number of studies have been conducted to evaluate the relationship between breastfeeding and development of allergies. Although there is some controversy, many authorities believe that breastfed infants are less likely to develop allergies, especially in the first year of life. The greatest benefit is for the genetically-at-risk infant whose parents are atopic. Breastfeeding seems to be more protective against asthma and bronchitis in the first year of life, whereas its effect on eczema is less clear. These benefits may be related to:

- A protective action of breast milk
- Exposure to foreign antigens in formulas
- Differences in intestinal morphology with different food sources

Cow's milk protein allergy is the most common food allergy in infants. The best protection against food allergy in infancy is breastfeeding and postponing the introduction to semi-solid foods until four to six months of age. Cow's milk protein can pass into breast milk and may initiate sensitization in predisposed infants. Parents of infants at genetic risk may be able to prevent milk allergy by avoiding milk products in the infant's diet and by limiting maternal milk intake while breastfeeding.

Nutritional Benefits

The nutrient composition of human milk is suited for human infants in various stages of growth and development. Human milk is all that is required to sustain growth and good nutritional status for the first four to six months of life in the infant of a well nourished mother who has optimal stores herself and maintains a nutritionally adequate diet. Most women produce breast milk of good volume and composition. Supplementary feedings provided to poorly nourished women may insure the volume and nutritional quality of their breast milk.

Colostrum, a carotenoid-rich fluid, is secreted up to 4 to 7 days after birth. Transitional milk is the term used to describe the milk in the postcolostral period. Milk is considered mature at 21 days postpartum. Additionally, the milk of women who deliver preterm infants is substantially different (more protein, sodium, chloride; lower lactose) from full-term mothers, and the time to transitional milk is longer (several weeks) for these women.

The content of mature human milk is different from cow's milk. Components that differ include:

- Protein
- Fat
- Carbohydrate
- Vitamins
- Minerals

Human milk contains about three times less protein than cow's milk; the major proteins found in breast milk are casein and lactalbumin. The curd of human milk is soft and flocculent, and the small curds are easily digested and tolerated by infants. The cholesterol content of human milk is higher than cow's milk, which may be beneficial in stimulating the development of enzymes necessary later for cholesterol degradation.

Exclusively breastfed infants clearly demonstrate differences in growth from formula-fed infants. The primary difference in growth is in the weight-to-length relationship; breastfed infants appear to be leaner than bottle fed infants. The relationship between breastfeeding and subsequent obesity has not been conclusively resolved. Small differences in linear growth between breast and bottle-fed infant boys has also been demonstrated. As current reference data for evaluating infant growth is based on formula-fed infants, it may appear to clinicians that breastfed infants' growth falters after two to three months. There is no association of these slower growth rates and lower caloric intakes with morbidity, activity level or behavioral development. The slower rate of weight gain in breastfed infants may be considered normal, but investigation into this phenomena continues.

Psychological Benefits
Maternal-infant bonding has been demonstrated to be related to close physical contact between the mother and infant during a sensitive period of time, most frequently believed to be within the first 24 hours post-delivery. The probability of a dysfunctional mother-child relationship may be increased in parents and children who do not experience this bonding. Close physical contact during the first hour post-delivery appears to be related to subsequent maternal attitudes and child rearing practices.

The breastfeeding experience may facilitate bonding through the more direct physical and biological relationship between the mother and infant.

Convenience and Economic Benefits
Breastfeeding may be more convenient for the mother than bottle feeding. If managed appropriately, breast milk is:

- Always ready
- At the right temperature
- Safe and sanitary

The cost of infant formula has risen in recent years and is greater than the cost of additional food required by the lactating woman. This difference in cost is:
- Variable
- Dependent upon dietary habits and preferences
- Of greater impact for low income families

Birth Spacing

Researchers now endorse full or nearly full breastfeeding as a viable method of birth control for mothers of full-term, normal infants in both developing and developed countries. In order for breastfeeding to be appropriate for a given individual, the following criteria must be noted:
- The mother must be fully or nearly fully breastfeeding
- The mother remains amenorrheic (non-inclusive of any bleeding prior to the 56th day postpartum)

Breastfeeding provides more than 98 percent protection from pregnancy in the first six months when these two conditions are met. Regular supplementation of the infant's diet may lead to the return of fertility due to decreased breast stimulation. The current recommendation to delay introduction of supplemental foods to the infant until four to six months supports the use of breastfeeding as a family planning method.

#2 Expression of Breast Milk

2. **Introduction**

Milk can be expressed by hand or with the aid of an electric or hand pump. Circumstances under which expression of breast milk is useful include:

- Easing breast engorgement
- Maintaining milk supply without a suckling infant (e.g., temporary discontinuation of nursing or when a newborn remains hospitalized and the mother desires to resume breastfeeding when the infant comes home)
- Appropriate management of nipple confusion
- Appropriate management of an infant who suckles poorly
- Frequent separation from an older infant (e.g., mother returning to work)

Assessment

Before recommending a method of breast milk expression, the circumstances requiring it need to be determined. Under different circumstances, it may be most appropriate to use:

- Hand-expression
- A hand pump
- An electric pump

Management

Regardless of what method is to be employed, expression of breast milk may be intimidating and awkward for some women. It is important for women to become comfortable with expression or pumping to integrate it successfully into their nursing experience. This is particularly important for women who desire to breastfeed exclusively, as short separations from their infants may occur, even if unplanned, and will be required of women returning to work.

The amount of milk that a woman is able to pump depends on the time of day, the level of nursing by the infant, and the time of the last infant feeding. Hand massage of the breasts prior to pumping will increase the volume of milk collected.

It is quite reasonable for a woman to build a surplus of milk she may use for occasional separations from the infant (see Section #3 for storage guidelines). This may be accomplished by adding a "pumping" session the same time each day into the nursing schedule. Many women find that they are able to pump larger quantities of milk in the morning. If separation from the infant is frequent, (e.g., a woman returning to work), she will need to pump milk more often (see Section #4).

Hand-Expression

When the mother is engorged, hand-expression is the best technique for relief. Since it is difficult for some women to hand-express a significant quantity of milk beyond the initial postpartum period, it may not be the preferred method in circumstances requiring frequent or prolonged expression. The appropriate technique for hand-expression is as follows:

- First, the mother needs to drain the milk reservoirs by positioning her thumb and first two fingers 1 to 1 1/2 inch behind the nipple, then pushing straight back into the chest wall. She should then release her fingers by rolling them forward (do not slide) towards the nipple. This motion of pushing, then

rolling forward should be repeated rhythmi-
cally, rotating around the breast to empty all
reservoirs
- Second, the mother should massage her
breasts to move the milk forward. Massage
from the chest wall towards the nipple, cir-
culating around the entire breast (see Figure 2.1)
- The draining and massage should be repeated until her breasts are soft enough for
the baby to nurse
- If breasts are very engorged, the use of
warm compresses or a warm shower can
bring the milk down more comfortably than
massage
- The best time to learn the skill of hand-
expression is during a nursing session when
"let down" has occurred and milk flows with
greater ease

Hand Pumps

If there is separation from the baby or cessation of nursing for short, infrequent, periods of
time, hand pumping is often the preferred method
of expressing breast milk.

The preferred hand pumps are cylindric. These
pumps are:
- Comfortable
- Inexpensive
- Able to be sterilized
- Efficient

These may be available at local retail stores;
however, in many parts of the country a medical
supply store may be the only source for breast
pumps. Follow the use and cleaning instructions
included with the pump.

"Bicycle Horn"-style pumps are not recommended. They can cause breast tissue damage and are not very effective. Breast milk collected with these pumps has been shown to carry significant bacterial contamination.

Electric Pumps

Electric pumps may be the best choice when there are long-term or frequent separations of mother and infant, such as:
- Hospitalization of the infant
- Prematurity
- Mother returning to work

Electric pumps may be available through a hospital, or they can be rented from a medical supplier. They work by simulating infant sucking. A vacuum is created around the nipple and, upon let-down, milk is discharged into a bottle or other container. Electric pumps empty the breasts most efficiently of all the pumps.

There are multiple manufacturers of electric breast pumps, though only a few are priced low enough for most women to consider purchasing. Features of electric pumps include the strength of the suction mechanism, automated versus manual control of the suction, the ability to "double-pump" (i.e., pump both breasts at one time), flexible versus hard flanges and conversion capabilities to manual, more portable pumps. Figures 2.2 and 2.3 illustrate examples of manual and electric pumps. Manufacturers/distributors of electric breast pumps include Medela (1-800-435-8316) and Ameda/Egnell (1-800-323-8750) and The Natural Choice Company (1-800-528-8880).

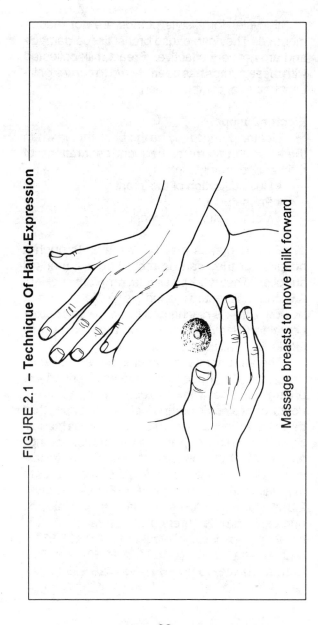

FIGURE 2.1 – Technique Of Hand-Expression

Massage breasts to move milk forward

26

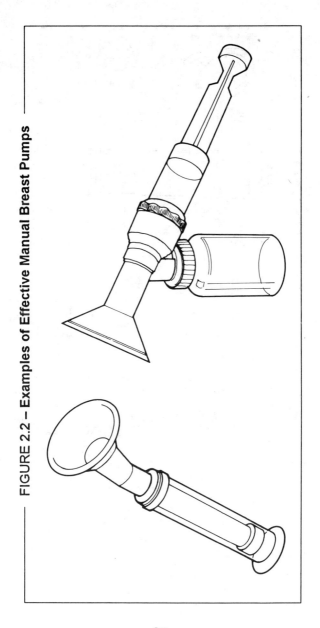

FIGURE 2.2 – Examples of Effective Manual Breast Pumps

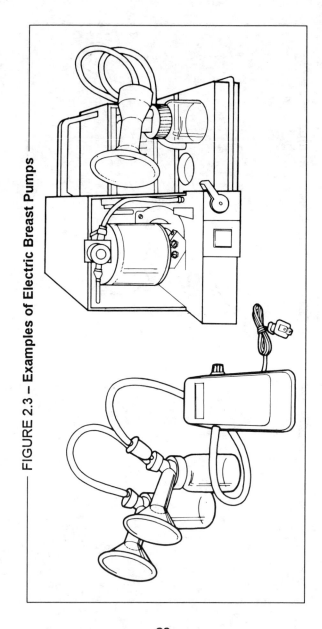

FIGURE 2.3 – Examples of Electric Breast Pumps

NOTES

#3 Storage of Breast Milk

Introduction

There are many instances when a woman may need to store breast milk for future use. When advising women on the storage of breast milk, specific issues need to be considered, including:

- Sanitation
- Shelf life
- Storage containers
- Storage temperature

Management

Appropriate handling and storage of breast milk will assure that the milk can be safely given to the baby at a later date.

Refrigeration

The following precautions should be observed when refrigerating breast milk:

- Clear glass or plastic bottles should be used
- If immediate refrigeration is not available, freshly pumped breast milk may be kept up to 6 hours at room temperature (66°-79°F)
- Refrigerated breast milk should be used within 48 hours

Freezing

Breast milk may be frozen for longer storage. The following precautions should be observed when freezing breast milk:

- Plastic Playtex nurser bags or a similar brand that is easy to use, sterile and safe should be sealed (with a twist tie or scotch tape, if not self-sealing) and dated

- Breast milk may be kept for three weeks in the freezing compartment of the refrigerator or three to six months in a deep freezer
- Frozen breast milk should be quick-thawed under cold running water and used promptly after defrosting
- Frozen breast milk should not be thawed at room temperature
- Frozen breast milk should not be thawed in a microwave
- Thawed breast milk should never be refrozen
- Fresh breast milk should not be added to already frozen milk, though small amounts of milk frozen separately can be combined after defrosting

#4 Nursing and Working

Introduction

Once a woman has made the decision to return to work, she needs some very specific information regarding the maintenance of breastfeeding. Many women are so anxious about their ability to nurse and work that it may influence their decision to initiate breastfeeding.

These women should be reassured that many mothers find that they can successfully manage both nursing and working. It is important not to let concerns about working and breastfeeding influence the decision to start nursing.

Factors associated with success in nursing and working include:
- Part-time employment
- The ability to pump and store breast milk at work
- Pumping or expressing breast milk frequently
- Older, better educated mothers
- Support from family
- Good maternal diet and increased fluid intake

Management

A woman who is interested in returning to work should be advised that she should wait to do so until lactation is fully established. This usually takes four to six weeks. Returning to work before this time and expecting to continue significant nursing is probably unrealistic. If the baby is four to six weeks old and lactation is established, the mother should be able to continue nursing and return to work.

About two weeks before returning to work the mother should:

- Learn to express and pump milk (see Section #2)
- Decide whether she is going to give the infant iron-fortified formula or stored, expressed breast milk when she cannot be with the infant for a feeding (see Section #3)
- Introduce the baby to a rubber nipple and have someone other than herself feed the baby
- Select clothing that facilitates pumping and/or nursing
- Select a child care helper who is supportive of breastfeeding

While at work, the mother should:

- Nurse just before leaving and as soon as returning from work, even if the infant has to be awakened to do so
- Go to her child or have him brought to her throughout the day to nurse, if possible. Lunch breaks may be the best time for this for many women
- Instruct the sitter not to feed the infant within one hour of the return time
- Provide the sitter with ample quantities of expressed breast milk to meet the infant's demands and to determine how much the infant will normally require
- Express or pump her breasts frequently (e.g., once mid-morning and once mid-afternoon). The milk can be saved if stored in a refrigerator (see Section #3)

The most common concern of working women who attempt to continue nursing is maintenance of an adequate milk supply. To avoid problems, the mother should:

- Make sure she pumps or expresses milk often during the day
- Nurse her baby as often as she can, eliminating bottle feedings as much as possible on weekends and at night when she is with the baby
- Drink plenty of fluids throughout the day
- Decrease her involvement with other activities and get enough rest
- Eat properly to insure adequate milk supply
- Be aware of and prepared for increased nursing demands of the infant during growth spurts

NOTES

#5 Maternal Support

Introduction

A woman with an inadequate support network will present to the health professional expressing anxiety regarding quantity or quality of her milk, a fussy infant or another seemingly unrelated problem.

Most women must have support to breastfeed successfully. Studies indicate that maternal support is the most influential factor affecting duration of breastfeeding. Members of a support network provide:

- Physical support
- Emotional support
- Psychological support

A woman requires physical support for maintenance of the home and help with any other children. She requires emotional support in the form of encouragement and positive reinforcement of her breastfeeding behaviors. She needs psychological support, i.e., someone who is sensitive to and understanding of her feelings about nursing. This support can be provided by one or a combination of a number of different individuals, including:

- The father
- The maternal or parental grandmother
- A female friend or sister
- The health care provider

The opinions and actions of these individuals, although they may not necessarily be supportive of breastfeeding, have an influence on the decisions and behavior of the mother. It is important to understand that the influence is not always positive.

Assessment

The health care provider must determine if there is someone that influences the mother's desire to nurse and her success in nursing. Research indicates that this person may vary among ethnic groups. In Anglo families, the father appears to have a significant impact on the nursing experience. In Hispanic families, the father is less likely to be involved in infant feeding practices, as they are managed by the mother and the maternal or paternal grandmother. For African American women, a sister or friend appears to be the advisor and confidant. When other individuals are not available to the mother, the health care provider seems to become the most significant source of support.

While it is not appropriate to apply these general observations carte blanche, it can be a beginning to understand the decisions made by the mother and a basis for eliciting assistance for her.

Careful and sensitive questioning of the mother may be necessary to determine:

- If she has anyone providing such support and who that individual is
- If anyone is discouraging her, in words or actions, from continuing to nurse

Since the influence of the father is often significant, it is important to understand his reaction to the nursing process. The feelings of a father to his partner who is nursing an infant may include:

- Pride
- Envy
- Inadequacy
- Jealousy

- Exclusion
- Discomfort
- Sexual anxiety or jealousy

Responses of the father to these and other possible emotions may include:
- Feelings of guilt
- Feelings of hostility
- Withdrawal
- Resentment
- Lack of support for breastfeeding

Management

The role of the health care provider is to:
- Provide information, reinforcement and support
- Help assure that the mother has other individuals supportive of her breastfeeding decision available for answering questions and providing reassurance and reinforcement
- Identify and counteract any possible negative influence the mother has been exposed to
- Enlist the participation of influential individuals in supporting the breastfeeding woman

This can be done by:
- Including influential individuals in any counseling, whenever possible
- Advising fathers, mothers or friends of their importance in the nursing experience
- Educating influential individuals about the benefits and mechanics of breastfeeding so they can provide the support needed

- Encouraging the new parents to find a reliable, trustworthy substitute caretaker for the infant so they may still enjoy times alone
- Respecting the importance of the marital relationship and recognizing the role each parent has
- Encouraging the mother to include the father in the nursing experience if he is non-supportive
- Educating the new parents about the appropriate use of expressed breast milk, which may be given to an older infant by others
- Assuring that the new parents understand that the first four to six weeks are the most demanding of the nursing experience and that the process will get easier with time
- Putting the mother in touch with any local breastfeeding support groups, e.g., La Leche League, lactation consultants or public health services
- Reinforcing the idea that, although the infant demands much of her time right now, it is important for the mother to maintain relationships with other adults as well
- Conducting community-based education (e.g., social sororities, church groups, mass media) to increase social support for breastfeeding

#6 Nutritional Requirements of Breastfeeding Women

Introduction

Food intake is a concern for breastfeeding women due primarily to its effect on the mother herself and in some instances on the infant. In well-nourished populations, the main dietary concern is to maintain the nutritional status of the mother, particularly maternal stores of calcium, magnesium, zinc, folate and vitamin B_6. It may also be important to assure adequate caloric intake, particularly among women interested in rapid weight loss. In poorly nourished women, inadequate diet may directly affect the quantity and quality of breast milk.

Lactation increases the requirements for 17 nutrients as well as for calories. The increase is even greater for lactating adolescents. Table 6.1 lists the Recommended Dietary Allowances (RDA) for lactating adolescents and adults.

An inadequate consumption of calories may result in a decreased supply of breast milk, especially in poorly nourished women. If the maternal diet is inadequate in water-soluble vitamins, the level of these vitamins in the breast milk will be lower. Also, the type of fat in the milk varies with the type of fat found in the diet.

The protein content of breast milk usually remains at a constant level as long as maternal stores are maintained. The calcium content of breast milk does not vary with the mother's intake, since calcium is mobilized from maternal stores when her dietary intake is inadequate. The caloric value of the milk also remains constant, as long as maternal resources are present.

The level of fat-soluble vitamins in breast milk is not greatly altered by the intake of the mother. However, if the maternal diet has been inadequate for some time, maternal stores of fat-soluble vitamins may be mobilized to assure adequate levels in breast milk. Vitamin B_6, vitamin D, iodine and selenium have been shown in breast milk at unusually high levels with infants' high intakes of breast milk. The significance of this is presently unknown.

It takes four to six hours for components or metabolites of a specific food to appear in the breast milk. Occasionally, specific foods ingested by the mother may flavor the milk or otherwise make it unacceptable to the infant. Allergens from foods that a mother consumes may enter her milk and promote an allergic reaction in a sensitive infant. Although identifying the offending food is fraught with difficulty, the mother may discontinue consumption of a suspected food to determine if the infant's allergic symptoms are alleviated. However, she should not eliminate major nutrient sources, and dietary counseling should be provided to assure long-term nutritional adequacy for her infant.

Assessment

In *Nutrition During Lactation*, the Institute of Medicine (IOM) advises that all lactating women be asked questions to determine if:

- The mother eats calcium-rich foods regularly
- Their diets contain vitamin D-fortified milk or cereal or there is exposure to ultraviolet light
- The mother eats fruits and vegetables regularly

- The mother is a complete vegetarian
- The mother restricts her food intake severely in an attempt to lose weight or treat a medical condition
- If there are circumstances that might interfere with their eating adequate diets (e.g., poverty, drug or alcohol abuse)

Management

The objective in managing the maternal diet is to assure that there is a sufficient supply of nutritionally complete breast milk to support a healthy, growing infant and that maternal nutrient stores are not depleted nor maternal tissues jeopardized.

The mother should be counseled to consume a variety of foods every day, including:
- Fruits and vegetables
- Whole-grain breads and cereals
- Calcium-rich dairy products
- Protein-rich foods such as meats, fish and legumes

Current dietary recommendations suggest:
- Nine servings of bread, cereal, rice and pasta (preferably some whole grains)
- Four servings of vegetables
- Three servings of fruits
- Three servings of milk and/or milk products
- Two to three servings of meat and protein alternatives

The IOM recommends emphasizing sources of nutrients most likely to be deficient in lactating women's diets. Essential nutrients and their sources include:

- Calcium found in milk, cheese, yogurt, fish with edible bones, tofu processed with calcium sulfate, bok choy, broccoli, kale, and collard, mustard and turnip greens
- Zinc, found in meat, poultry, seafood, eggs, seeds, legumes, yogurt, and whole grains
- Magnesium, found in nuts, seeds, legumes, whole grains, green vegetables, scallops and oysters
- Vitamin B_6, found in bananas, poultry, meat, fish, potatoes, sweet potatoes, spinach, prunes, watermelon, some legumes, fortified cereals and nuts
- Folate, found in leafy vegetables, fruit, liver, green beans, fortified cereals, legumes and whole grain cereals

The mother should be counseled:
- That the energy (caloric) requirements for breastfeeding are greater than the energy requirements of pregnancy. It is assumed that some of the fat deposited in pregnancy will be used to support lactation; however, dietary energy intakes generally increase while a woman is lactating. The current RDA in support of lactation is 500 kcal/day above the caloric intake recommended for non-lactating women
- That many, but not all, women lose weight while breastfeeding — generally a pound or two a month. Weight loss in itself is not believed to affect lactation adversely if a woman is well nourished, as long as she consumes a nutritionally adequate diet and loses at an acceptable rate. Women should not restrict their energy intake at all in the first few weeks postpartum. After this, an

intake greater than 1800 kcal/day is recommended for all women. Higher minimum intakes are recommended for underweight women

- To supplement her diet with multivitamin preparations commensurate with the RDA if her diet is consistently inadequate in particular nutrients (e.g., 600 mg elemental calcium/day taken with meals for women who avoid dairy products). This should be based on individualized dietary assessment and counseling
- That if she is a total vegetarian, she should receive specific nutritional guidance from a nutritionist or dietitian and include a regular source of vitamin B_{12}, such as a special food product or 2.6 micrograms of supplemental vitamin B_{12} daily. Vitamin B_{12}, deficiency has been reported in a breastfed infant of a strict vegetarian
- That fluid intake should be governed by thirst
- That she need not routinely avoid any particular foods or spices. However, if a certain food or spice produces a reaction in the infant and if it can be identified, it may be omitted from her diet. Elimination of all suspected foods for at least two weeks, followed by reintroduction of the omitted foods one by one until symptoms reappear, may help in identification of offending foods. The counselor should make sure the mother's diet remains nutritionally adequate by suggesting alternatives, if necessary

TABLE 6.1 — Recommended Dietary Allowances For Lactating Females

Nutrient	First 6 Months	Second 6 Months
Protein (g)	65	62
Vitamin A (mcg RE)	1300	1200
Vitamin D (mcg)	10	10
Vitamin E (mg TE)	12	11
Vitamin C (mg)	95	90
Vitamin K (mcg)	65	65
Thiamin (mg)	1.6	1.6
Riboflavin (mg)	1.8	1.7
Niacin (mg NE)	20	20
Vitamin B_6 (mg)	2.1	2.1
Folacin (mcg)	280	260
Vitamin B_{12} (mcg)	2.6	2.6
Calcium (mg)	1200	1200
Phosphorus (mg)	1200	1200
Magnesium (mg)	355	340
Iron (mg)	15	15
Zinc (mg)	19	16
Iodine (mcg)	200	200
Selenium (mcg)	75	75
Energy (Kcal)*	2700	2700

* Recommendations for energy intake are average energy allowances for women of average body size who engage in moderate activity and should be adjusted for any differences.

Recommended Dietary Allowances, National Academy Press, 1989.

#7 Medications and Breast Milk

Introduction

Almost any ingested medication that can enter the blood stream of a lactating woman can enter breast milk. The issue of whether to discontinue nursing while the mother is taking specific medications is frequently debated, and numerous articles on the subject of drugs in breast milk have been written. However, most articles are based on a combination of theoretical concerns and single-case reports infrequently validated by critical pharmacological study. The lack of reliable data and the many variables that determine drug levels in the breastfed infant make decisions difficult.

7.
All unnecessary medications should be avoided by nursing mothers, and any required medications should be used carefully and in moderation. However, it is generally unnecessary for a nursing mother to discontinue breastfeeding while taking medications, because most prescribed medications are:

- Of low toxicity
- Only prescribed for short periods of time
- Present in lower concentrations in breast milk than in maternal plasma
- Present in undetectable or at least non-toxic levels in breast milk

Management of Medications

The basic question for the health care provider managing a nursing woman is whether the risk to the infant exposed to a medication is greater than the benefits of his being breastfed. It is usually inappropriate to discontinue breastfeeding, since the risks are frequently minimal. If the medication is normally considered safe to prescribe to an infant, it is probably safe to prescribe to the nursing mother.

The concentration of maternal medications in breast milk is usually lowest one hour prior to the next scheduled dose. Infant exposure to maternal medication can be minimized by:

- Scheduling drug administration shortly after the nursing session
- Prolonging the nursing interval prior to the next feeding
- Avoiding long-acting forms of a drug

Over-the-Counter Drugs

Certain over-the-counter drugs, if used in moderation, should have no significant effect on the baby. Examples of these drugs include:

- Acetaminophen
- Ibuprofen
- Cough medicines
- Antacids
- Antihistamines/decongestants

Oral Contraceptives

Oral contraceptives (OCs) are a relative contraindication for breastfeeding mothers. OCs have been reported to decrease production and alter the quality of breast milk. Their effect on the infant is unknown. However, the majority of the available data is based on steroid dosages infrequently prescribed in current practice, and the reported changes in breast milk composition are minimal. The woman's circumstances and risk of pregnancy must be weighed against the possible risks associated with OCs and breastfeeding. If OCs are used, they should contain the lowest possible doses of estrogen and progesterone.

Alcohol

Alcohol use may be harmful for the nursing infant. Some studies suggest that modest amounts of alcohol have a slight but detrimental effect on motor development. Infants have also been found to consume less breast milk after their mothers' have taken even small quantities of alcoholic beverages. Excessive alcohol use decreases the milk-ejection reflex and has produced effects on infants such as:

- Failure to thrive
- Hypoglycemia
- Pseudo-Cushing's syndrome

Mothers should be advised to limit or discontinue drinking of alcoholic beverages while breastfeeding.

Marijuana

The effects of maternal use of marijuana on the infant have not been fully investigated. However, because of the long half-life of THC and subsequent potential for accumulation with chronic use, some researchers feel that there is potential for harm to the infant. Mothers should be advised against the use of marijuana.

Cocaine

There are a limited number of reports on maternal use of cocaine and subsequent intoxication by a breastfeeding infant. Mothers should be advised regarding the hazards of cocaine use and its potential effects on the developing infant and should be advised to discontinue its use.

Clinical signs of cocaine intoxication in the infant include:

- Rapid heart rate
- Rapid respiration
- Hypertension
- Irritability
- Tremulousness

Nicotine

Infants whose mothers smoke have increased rates of respiratory infections. Additionally, women who smoke are more likely to discontinue breastfeeding within the first three months. Breast-fed infants of smoking women are exposed to constituents of smoke as passive smokers and through breast milk.

Nicotine levels reached when the mother smokes in excess of one pack of cigarettes per day may cause effects on the infant such as:

- Restlessness
- Diarrhea
- Vomiting
- Tachycardia
- Colic or excessive crying

Nicotine is excreted in breast milk in high concentrations. The level of health risk posed to a breastfed infant whose mother smokes is unknown. It is ill advised to suggest to mothers ways to accommodate any maternal smoking (e.g., delaying feedings or cutting down on smoking). Mothers must be advised to discontinue cigarette smoking throughout lactation.

Caffeine

Mothers should be advised to drink coffee and caffeinated colas only in moderation while breastfeeding or to drink decaffeinated varieties of beverages, since caffeine:

- Is excreted into breast milk with relative ease
- Does accumulate in the infant
- May cause irritability and poor sleeping in the infant

Summary

A breastfeeding mother should be advised to:
- Use over-the-counter medications in moderation only
- Advise her physician that she is breastfeeding prior to obtaining any prescription medication
- Observe the infant for signs and symptoms of possible reactions to medications she is taking
- Discontinue cigarette smoking

Contraindicated Medications

According to the American Academy of Pediatrics, the following medications are contraindicated in breastfeeding:
- Bromocriptine
- Cyclophosphamide
- Cyclosporine
- Doxorubicin
- Ergotamine
- Lithium
- Methotrexate
- Phenindione
- Radioactive pharmaceuticals
- Sulfonamides (during first month)

Additionally, the following drugs of abuse are contraindicated:

- Amphetamines
- Cocaine
- Heroin
- Marijuana
- Nicotine (smoking)
- Phencyclidine (PCP)

#8 Cesarean Delivery

Introduction

Some women erroneously believe that they will not be able to nurse if they have a cesarean delivery. The mechanisms of lactation are not affected by the method of delivery or by the surgical procedure of cesarean section.

However, women who have had a cesarean delivery may experience unique difficulties in initiating breastfeeding. Physical pain, effects of pain medication on the mother's state of consciousness and her inability to independently access and position the infant for nursing are issues that must be managed. Some women who have had a cesarean delivery are disappointed in their birthing experience. It is especially rewarding to assist these women in initiating and maintaining a successful nursing experience.

8.

Management

Women who have had a cesarean delivery are equally as capable of nursing as women who have had a vaginal delivery. In the immediate post-delivery period, the woman may be drowsy from anesthesia and distracted by pain. Nursing staff will need to be involved in the early nursing sessions and frequently may need to help initiate this activity.

When nursing the baby, the mother will need help in finding a comfortable position to facilitate breastfeeding. One recommended position is with the mother sitting up with pillows to support her head, shoulders, arms, as well as across her abdomen to protect her incision and help support the baby. The mother's feet should be propped so that her knees are comfortably raised. Since the mother is post-surgical, the knee gatch in a hospital bed should not be raised. The baby can be held so that he is lying on his side on the pillow across the mother's abdomen or in a "football hold" position with his head in her hand and his feet under her arm.

Another position is with the mother lying on her side, with pillows to support her head, shoulders, back and knees (see Figure 8.1). The baby can be laid on his side in the crook of the mother's arm.

The health care professional should counsel the mother that:

- If she has been given a general anesthesia, her baby may be sleepier and spit up more frequently than a baby born vaginally
- She should take the pain medication prescribed by her doctor. The medication will not affect the baby during the first few days of nursing and the mother needs to be comfortable enough to nurse and bond with her baby
- She will require additional rest and may need to find someone who can help her when she first comes home from the hospital

FIGURE 8.1 – Side-by-Side Position

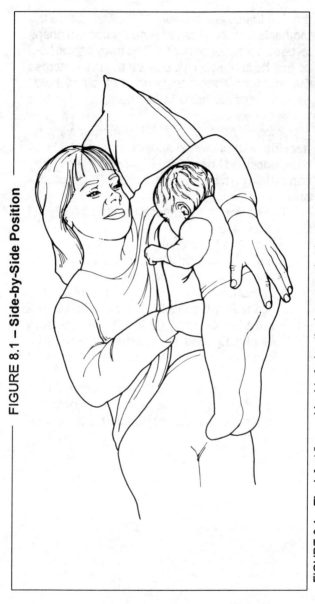

FIGURE 8.1 – The infant lies on his side facing the breast so that he does not need to turn his head to nurse.

NOTES

#9 Nursing Twins

Introduction

Many people feel that breastfeeding twins presents overwhelming problems and physiologic demands on the mother. This is not necessarily true, and the arguments for nursing twins are as strong as arguments for nursing single babies.

A mother who is nursing twins needs a thorough understanding of the techniques of nursing and of the law of supply and demand. If the mother nurses often on demand, she will have enough milk for both babies. Nursing twins presents a special but manageable situation.

Management

Special considerations in the management of nursing twins include:
- Scheduling
- Use of supplements
- Positioning
- Physiological demand on the mother

9.

Scheduling

As with other infants, twins need to be able to nurse on demand. A rigid nursing schedule is an unrealistic expectation during the first few weeks. The mother can work towards a regular schedule but needs to be aware that, to ensure an adequate milk supply, the babies will have to nurse often.

The two babies may have different nursing needs. However, the mother should be encouraged to nurse the babies simultaneously whenever possible.

The mother should be advised:
- To feed the infants on demand

- That it will probably not be possible to maintain a regular feeding schedule during the first few weeks
- To nurse the infants simultaneously whenever possible, since this will facilitate establishing a routine schedule as the infants get older
- That learning to nurse the twins simultaneously may take a little patience but that the mother will become skillful with practice

Supplements

If the mother nurses often on demand, she will have an adequate milk supply and will not need to supplement breastfeeding. The mother should be advised not to supplement the breast milk within the first four to six weeks. However, because of the twins' added demands on the mother's time, she may choose to provide supplemental feeding later.

The mother should be advised:

- Not to supplement breastfeeding until the babies are four to six weeks old. However, if the mother is discouraged and is considering termination of nursing, supplements may be introduced earlier (two to three weeks)
- That giving occasional formula on an irregular basis after the first four to six weeks is appropriate
- Not to give supplemental formula on a regular basis as this may decrease her milk supply

Positioning

Positioning twins requires special techniques. Possible positions include:

- Holding both babies in the regular nursing position, their legs beside each other or one's legs on top of the other's (see Figure 9.1)

- Placing both babies in the "football hold," their heads in the mother's hands and their feet under the mother's arm (see Figure 9.2)
- Holding one baby in the regular nursing position and the other in a "football hold" (see Figure 9.3)
- Lying down with one baby beside the mother and the other across her body
- Using pillows to help support the babies and the mother's arms

Mothers are often concerned about whether it is important to alternate breasts between the infants. The mother should be advised that:
- When the infants are young, she should offer both breasts to both infants
- As they get older, the infants may develop a preference for one breast. This presents no problem as each breast's milk supply will meet the baby's needs
- There is no need for the mother to be overly concerned about this issue; reassurance may be necessary

Physiologic Demand On The Mother
Nursing mothers of twins have increased physiological needs. The mother should be advised that:
- She should consume additional food to prevent adverse weight loss and to ensure an adequate milk supply
- Her diet should be adequate in all nutrients
- Her fluid intake should be governed by thirst
- She should get adequate rest

FIGURE 9.1 — **Regular Position for Nursing Twins**

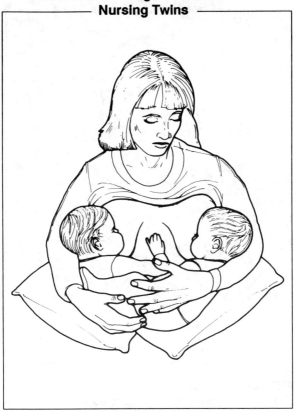

FIGURE 9.1 — Holding both babies in regular nursing position, their legs beside each other or one's legs on top of the other.

FIGURE 9.2 — **"Football Hold" Position for Nursing Twins**

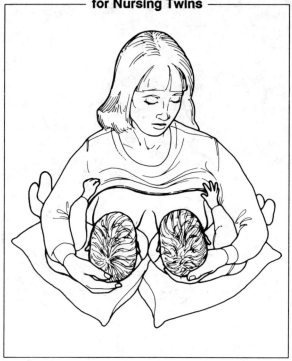

FIGURE 9.2 — Both babies placed in the "football hold," their heads in the mother's hands and their feet under the mother's arms.

FIGURE 9.3 — **Regular and "Football" Position for Nursing Twins**

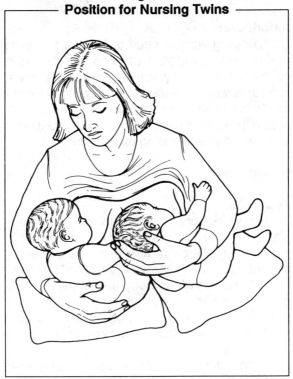

FIGURE 9.3 — Holding one baby in a regular position and the other in a "football hold."

#10 Nursing Techniques

Introduction

Lactating women need to have a thorough understanding of the basic techniques of nursing to initiate successfully, to maintain and to prevent problems with breastfeeding. Correct positioning, frequent nursing and good nipple and breast care will help both the mother and the infant have a satisfying breastfeeding experience.

Management

Positioning

Proper positioning will help the infant suck effectively, with his jaws compressing the area behind the nipple on the areola. It will also prevent sore nipples, which are usually caused by incorrect positioning of the baby at the breast. The mother should be advised that:

- The infant should be lying on his side facing the breast so that he does not need to turn his head to nurse
- The infant should be held at the same level as the breast. This can be managed in the traditional nursing position (see Figure 10.1) with his head supported in the crook of the mother's arm and his buttocks supported by the mother's hand or in the "football hold" position (see Figure 10.2) with the mother holding the baby's head in her hand and his legs extending under her arm
- The baby's lower arm should be around the mother's waist, not pinned between baby and mother

10.

- The mother should support her breast between her thumb and hand with the fingers
  of her hand supporting the breast. Thumb
  and fingers should be well back from the
  areola (see Figure 10.3)
- The mother should touch the baby's lips
  lightly with her nipple until he opens his
  mouth wide
- When the baby' mouth is open wide, the
  mother should draw the baby in so that he
  grasps the area behind the nipple on the
  areola
- The mother can indent her breast with her
  thumb to give air space to the baby's nose,
  if necessary
- To break suction, the mother should insert
  her finger into the corner of the infant's
  mouth

Nursing Schedule
   Early and frequent nursing will ensure an adequate milk supply, satisfy the infant and avoid
problems such as engorgement, plugged ducts
and mastitis. The mother should be advised:
- To nurse within the first hour after the baby
  is born
- To nurse on demand, at least every one and
  one half to three hours
- To nurse 10 to 15 minutes on each breast or
  until the baby seems satisfied
- To have the baby nurse from both breasts at
  each feeding
- That lactation works by the law of supply
  and demand. The more often she nurses,
  the more milk she will have if the baby is
  suckling well

Nipple and Breast Care

Basic nipple and breast care will help prevent soreness and infection. The mother should be advised to:

- Wear a good supportive bra that fits comfortably and does not bind
- Avoid use of plastic bra liners, pads or anything that keeps air from the nipple
- Air-dry nipples after feeding
- Avoid use of soap or alcohol on nipples
- Avoid use of breast creams that must be washed off

FIGURE 10.1 — **Traditional Nursing Position**

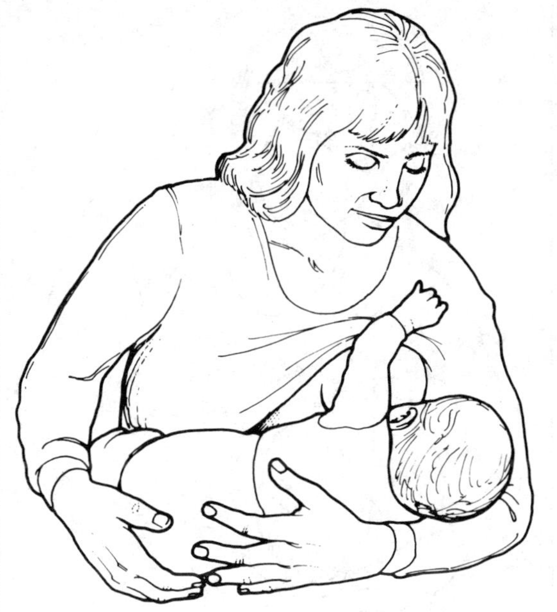

FIGURE 10.1 – Traditional position with the baby's head supported in the crook of the mother's arm, his arm around the mother's waist (not pinned between the mother and baby) and his buttocks supported by the mother's hand.

FIGURE 10.2 – Nursing Baby in "Football Hold" Position

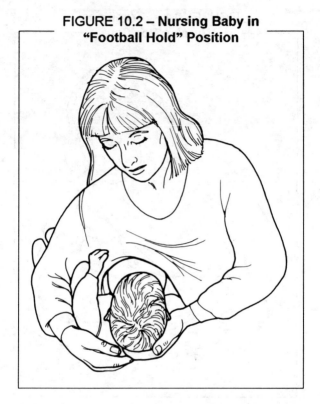

FIGURE 10.2 – The "football hold" with the mother holding the baby's head in one hand. The infant's legs are extended under the mother's arm.

FIGURE 10.3 – **Grasping the Breast**

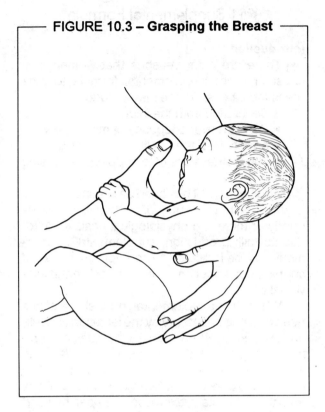

FIGURE 10.3 – The mother supports the breast between thumb and hand with the fingers of her hand supporting the breast while also pulling the baby in close so that he grasps the area behind the nipple on the areola.

#11 Supplemental Formula

Introduction

There are many reasons that women may consider giving supplemental formula to their breastfed infants. These may include:

- Separation from the infant
- Concern over adequacy of milk supply
- Anxiety over the quality of breast milk
- The mother's desire to supplement nursing

Additionally, if it has been determined that the infant is "nipple confused," otherwise suckles poorly or there is a physiological basis for inadequate milk production, supplemental nourishment may be indicated. The appropriate use of supplemental nourishment depends on the individual case.

Whenever supplemental nourishment has been deemed necessary by the lactation consultant or specialized health care provider, the preferred supplemental nourishment to provide is the mother's expressed breast milk. If the mother is returning to work or is facing frequent separations from the older infant, expressed milk can be used as well. Commercial formula may also be used in the latter case if the mother prefers or if she is not able to pump her breasts.

Assessment

If the mother questions the health care provider about the use of infant formula, it is extremely important for the provider to have a complete understanding of the origin of the request. The provider should discuss the request with the mother to determine if she:

- Is concerned about the quantity of breast milk
- Is anxious about the quality of breast milk
- Has been or will be separated from her infant
- Desires to have more separation from her infant and wants to supplement with formula

The health care provider may be the initiator of the topic of supplemental nourishment if it has been determined that:
- The infant is "nipple confused" (see Section #25)
- The infant exhibits flutter or negative sucking (see Section #25)
- Inadequate mammary glandular tissue syndrome has been diagnosed (see Section #16)

Management

It is important first to determine whether supplemental nourishment:
- Is necessary
- Will jeopardize the success of the breastfeeding experience
- Can be initiated successfully without premature weaning neither requested nor desired by the mother

Times when supplemental nourishment is not necessary and in fact will jeopardize the establishment of lactation generally occur within the first six weeks postpartum and include:
- The mother inaccurately feeling she has an inadequate milk supply

- The mother being unduly anxious about the quality of her breast milk
- The mother desiring supplementation before lactation is established

The first two of these problems should be managed as described in Sections #16 and #17.

Maternal Desire For Supplementation Prior
To Lactation Being Established

Any introduction of formula prior to the establishment of lactation (generally four to six weeks) will result in a decrease in milk production. The mother should be advised:

- To delay supplementation until lactation is established if she desires to continue nursing to any significant degree
- To increase the frequency of nursing sessions if she feels the infant is not receiving enough milk
- That her body's response to the increased sucking will be an increased milk production
- That the chances she will have a successful nursing experience will be greater if she delays supplementation
- That she may plan on supplementing as needed after this critical period has passed

Cases when supplemental nourishment may be necessary but must be managed carefully so as to not result in undesired weaning include:

- Effective management of an infant who exhibits nipple confusion
- Effective management of an infant exhibiting negative or flutter sucking

- Effective management of the nursing dyad when the mother and infant are separated while the infant is still less than six weeks old (e.g., hospitalization)

Managing Supplementation Of An Infant Exhibiting Nipple Confusion Or Poor Suckling

Emptying the breasts thoroughly is critical in managing nipple confusion or poor suckling. If the mother is successful at pumping or expressing breast milk and sanitary storage facilities are available, there is no reason not to provide this milk to the infant and there are many reasons to do so. When an efficient, manageable method of emptying the breasts (see Section #2) or sanitary method of breast milk storage (see Section #3) is not available to the mother, an iron-fortified, milk-based infant formula (soy-based if the infant has demonstrated cow milk allergy or intolerance) should be provided to the infant.

The key factor in managing the supplementation in these instances is that the feeding:
- Be on the breast
- Utilize a device such as a Lact-Aid or Supplemental Nutrition System (see Figure 11.1)

This will "teach the infant" how to nurse successfully and provide nourishment other than the breast milk the infant is obtaining.

It would also be appropriate to use either cup or spoon feedings for this period of time; however, this does not offer the advantage of assisting the infant in nursing. It is critical that a bottle with an artificial nipple not be used in these cases, as it is likely to exacerbate the original problem.

When Lact-Aid, Supplemental Nutrition System or cup or spoon feeding is necessary, careful instruction on the expression of breast milk is essential, regardless of whether the expressed milk will be fed to the infant. Inadequate emptying of the breasts at these times will result in involution of mammary tissue and cessation or reduction of milk production rendering the mother incapable of nursing.

The health care worker must supply the mother with a means for successfully emptying her breasts, including:

- Access to and proficiency in using manual or electric breast pumps
- Demonstrating proficiency at manual breast milk expression

Early Separation From The Infant

When the mother and infant are separated, as in hospitalization, the method of feeding the infant should be decided jointly by the physician, nurse and mother, taking into account the mother's desire for the method of feeding upon discharge of the infant. It is likely that full nursing will not be possible while the infant is hospitalized. Preferably some of the feedings will be of expressed milk administered without the use of an artificial nipple. In any case, if the mother desires to assume nursing upon the infant's arrival at home, she must pump her breasts routinely to keep producing milk. If this does not occur, the production of milk will cease.

Maternal Desire Or Need To
Supplement Nursing An Older Infant

Although its benefits are most pronounced when breastfeeding is exclusive, many women choose to supplement nursing to accommodate their modern lifestyles. The greatest chance for successfully instituting supplemental feedings of commercial formula without resulting in premature weaning is when lactation is fully established, generally not prior to four to six weeks postpartum. It is critically important that:

- Lactation is established prior to initiation
- The mother understands that supplementation will result in decreased milk production and decreased protective benefits

Inadequate Mammary Glandular Tissue Syndrome

When inadequate glandular development is diagnosed, supplemental feedings of a commercial formula will be necessary. The mother should be advised that:

- She may continue nursing
- To prevent nipple confusion, she should use Lact-Aid to increase nourishment provided during the nursing session while the infant is young
- She may choose to offer a bottle of formula to an older infant
- Formula should be offered at the end of the nursing session

In The Event Of Supplementation

If supplementation is initiated under any circumstances, the use of breastfeeding as a method of birth spacing will probably be inadequate. The woman should be advised to choose an alternate method of birth control through her medical care provider.

FIGURE 11.1 – **Medical Supplemental Nutrition System**

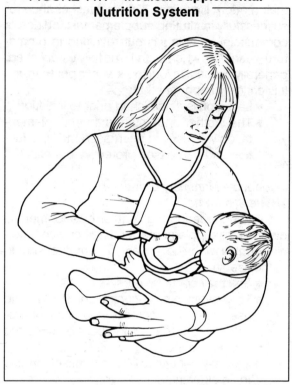

FIGURE 11.1 – Medical supplemental nutrition system used to provide supplemental formula simultaneously while breastfeeding.

#12 Supplemental Water

Introduction

Young infants do not need supplemental water while nursing. Breast milk is 87 percent water and provides all the water the baby requires.

Anything given to the infant with a rubber nipple can cause "nipple confusion" and should be discouraged. The flow of fluid through rubber nipples requires a different sucking action and less effort by the infant than sucking from the breast. This difference in sucking action and liquid flow confuses and frustrates the young infant, causing difficulty for both mother and infant.

Management

Water should not be given to an infant less than six weeks old unless given through a dropper. The health care provider should explain the "nipple confusion" concept to the mother (see Section #25).

The provider also should advise the mother that breast milk provides adequate fluid for the baby, even in hot weather.

Some physicians order water for jaundiced babies. However, current studies indicate that extra water does not affect the course of physiological jaundice and is not necessary (see Section #28).

12.

NOTES

#13 Pacifiers

Introduction

The use of a pacifier is not generally recommended for infants less than three weeks of age as any rubber nipple can cause "nipple confusion" (see Section #25). However, for older infants and under certain circumstances, judicious use of a pacifier is probably not harmful.

Assessment

Inappropriate use of a pacifier is indicated if:
- The infant is less than three weeks of age
- The mother is using a pacifier as a substitute for a feeding

Appropriate circumstances under which limited use of a pacifier can be helpful are:
- If the mother's nipples are extremely sore or cracked and she is limiting nursing time to 10 minutes on each side (see Section #18)
- If the mother is nursing twins (see Section #9)
- If the mother and baby are in a public situation where she feels uncomfortable nursing

Management

The mother needs to understand the appropriate uses of a pacifier. She should be counseled that:
- Pacifiers should not be used for an infant less than three weeks of age
- The baby needs to nurse every one and one half to three hours

13.

- She should not limit nursing time except under unusual circumstances
- The baby needs to be held, and the mother should hold and comfort him whenever possible (see Section #23)

#14 Breast and Nipple Shields

Introduction

Breast and nipple shields and their uses are commonly misunderstood. A breast shield is used to draw out an inverted nipple and is worn prenatally or between nursings. Breast shields are effective when they are worn correctly.

Nipple shields are promoted as providing protection for the mother's nipples or as facilitating infant sucking. However, nipple shields interfere with the successful initiation and maintenance of breastfeeding and should not be used.

Management

Breast Shields

Breast shields are sometimes referred to as "Woolrich Shields," after the original model or "milk cups." They are made of clear, hard, light weight plastic. Each shield has two parts: one part fits directly over the breast and has an opening for the nipple; another part, the cover, protects the emerging nipple from the mother's clothes. The purpose of breast shields is to draw out an inverted nipple. If the mother has inverted nipples and is using a breast shield or "milk cup," she should be advised to:

- Wear the cup under her bra for short periods of time and gradually work up to eight to 10 hours a day during the last months of pregnancy
- Wear the cup postnatally for short periods of time between nursing sessions

14.

- Be sure to remove the cup often to allow air circulation to reach the nipple. There are varieties of shields available which have multiple air holes to promote circulation of air around the nipple
- Discard any milk that collects in the cup as it may not be sterile

Nipple Shields

Nipple shields are rubber nipples that are designed to fit on the mother's breast over her nipples. They are used in the mistaken belief that they will protect and relieve sore nipples or that they will facilitate the infant's sucking. Actually, they can exacerbate nipple soreness or tenderness. They can also cause "nipple confusion", and it can be difficult to wean the infant off the shield. Both the thicker rubber "Mexican Hat" model and a new model made of thin silicone have been shown significantly to reduce the amount of milk made available to the infant.

The mother should be advised not to use nipple shields. There are other techniques for managing sore nipples (see Section #18) or facilitating infant suckling (see Section #25) that are more helpful and do not have the risks of using nipple shields. If the mother has been using nipple shields and the baby has become dependent on them, the mother needs to be helped to wean the baby off the shields. Alternatives to use of the shield to initiate breastfeeding and to wean the baby back to the bare breast include:

- Running ice lightly around the nipple to help it stand out
- Rolling the nipple between thumb and forefinger to elongate flat nipples

- Using a breast pump for a short while to draw out nipple
- Using breast shields between nursing sessions

See management of nipple confusion (Section #25.)

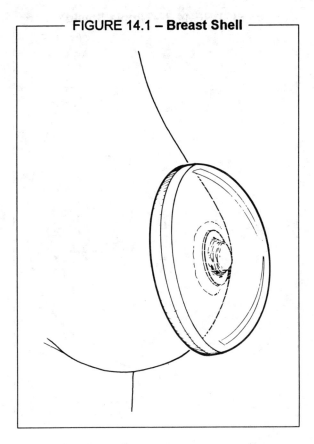

FIGURE 14.1 – **Breast Shell**

FIGURE 14.1 – The purpose of breast shields (shells) is to draw out an inverted nipple and protect the nipple from abrasion.

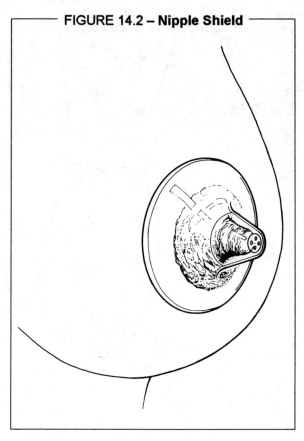

FIGURE 14.2 – Nipple Shield

FIGURE 14.2 – Nipple shields are not recommended for use by breastfeeding mothers.

NOTES

#15 Supplements and Addition of Other Food To Infant's Diet

Introduction

The timing of the addition of other foods to a breastfeeding infant's diet is important. Many mothers introduce other foods when the infant is very young. This practice should be discouraged to prevent:

- A decreased milk supply
- Overfeeding
- Development of food allergies
- Inappropriate feeding practices

Management

The mother should be advised not to introduce foods other than breast milk or formula until the infant is approximately four to six months of age.

The breastfeeding mother should be advised that:

- Any supplemental food introduced before four to six weeks will inhibit the establishment of lactation
- The young infant's immature gastrointestinal tract allows passage of macromolecules found in solid food into the blood stream, increasing the probability of future food allergies
- Early introduction of solid foods may increase the possibility of obesity in the infant
- The infant will display developmental readiness for solid foods by leaning forward to indicate an interest in food and pulling away if disinterested (normally between four to six months)

15.

- The infant needs supplemental feedings by four to six months of age to ensure adequate intake of iron
- Any supplemental food introduced at any age will decrease the mother's milk supply due to decreased infant demand

If the infant is ready for solid foods, the mother should be instructed to:
- Nurse the baby first
- Put food on a small spoon
- Start with a small amount of food
- Stop feeding when the baby indicates he has had enough
- Introduce one new food every four to five days
- Introduce a variety of foods so that, by the time the baby is eight months old, he is eating:
  - Cereal
  - Fruits
  - Vegetables
  - Meat
  - Milk products

Use of Nutritional Supplements

Nutritional supplements may be required for breastfed infants under certain circumstances. Supplementary fluoride, iron, vitamin D and zinc are sometimes indicated. Fluoride supplementation is needed if household water levels are less than .3 ppm; vitamin D supplementation may be appropriate for infants with low exposure to sunlight (7.0 micrograms/day); and supplemental iron should be provided if a food source is not being regularly consumed by the infant. The need for zinc supplementation remains controversial.

Maternal Problems	Inadequate Milk Supply	16.
	Anxiety Regarding Quality of Breast Milk	17.
	Sore Nipples	18.
	Sore Breasts (Engorgement)	19.
	Mastitis	20.
	Leaking Breasts	21.
	Maternal Illness	22.
Infant Problems	Fussy Infant	23.
	Sleepy Infant	24.
	Breast Refusal (Poor Suckling)	25.
	Infant Diarrhea	26.
	Infant Constipation	27.
	Jaundice	28.
	Thrush	29.
	Breast Preference	30.

#16 Inadequate Milk Supply

Introduction

Many breastfeeding women complain that:
- They do not have enough milk
- They are "drying up"
- The baby is not getting enough milk

It is important to acknowledge the mother's concern about the adequacy of her milk supply. Assessments must be made to determine if:
- The infant is displaying the classic signs of an inadequate milk supply
- Mother is feeding frequently enough
- Appropriate nursing techniques are being utilized

Occasionally, there is a physiological basis for inadequate milk production. These instances are rare and require a medical diagnosis.

Inadequate milk supply is the most common reason women give for discontinuing breastfeeding. In the absence of indications that the mother's milk supply could be insufficient, her perception of inadequate milk supply:
- Is termed "Insufficient Milk Syndrome" and is often due to a lack of knowledge or misinformation regarding breastfeeding
- Is exacerbated by a lack of a maternal support network
- Has serious implications for the maintenance of breastfeeding
- Hastens the onset of a true inadequacy of milk since mothers often give supplementary feedings to the infant or prolong the intervals between feedings

- May occasionally indicate that the mother would prefer not to breastfeed
- Can be overwhelming for the isolated breastfeeding mother

Assessment

To provide appropriate counseling and intervention, it must first be determined whether the baby is receiving enough breast milk.

The following signs generally indicate an adequate milk supply:

- The baby has an age-appropriate stooling pattern (i.e., newborns stool frequently, whereas older infants may go several days without stooling) and six to eight wet diapers a day
- The baby is happy and vigorous while awake
- The baby exhibits age-appropriate sleep patterns
- The baby has regained birth weight by two to three weeks and continues to gain $1/2$ to 1 ounce per day

INADEQUATE MILK

If the infant is not receiving an adequate amount of milk, the problem may be caused by improper nursing technique, maternal anxiety or improper maternal and infant diet. Only rarely is there a medical problem that adversely affects milk production.

Improper Nursing Technique

Improper nursing technique is indicated when:

- The mother is not nursing on demand every one and one-half to three hours

- Feedings are unnecessarily limited in length or are less than 10 to 15 minutes
- The baby is not nursing from both breasts at each feeding
- The baby is not grasping the areola and nursing effectively
- The baby exhibits "negative flutter" sucking or is sucking his own tongue or lower lip (see Section #25)

Maternal Anxiety

Maternal anxiety is indicated when the mother:
- Is not comfortable or relaxed while nursing
- States that she is unable to perform her domestic chores or she is not receiving enough help at home
- Is socially isolated, has few friends and her mother or father is not available to her
- States she is in a stressful environment

Improper Maternal and Infant Diet

Improper maternal and infant diet may be indicated when:
- The mother admits to not eating properly or to not drinking sufficient fluids
- A dietary assessment of the mother reveals poor intake of specific foods or nutrients
- The infant is eating solid foods prior to four months of age
- An infant less than six weeks of age is receiving supplemental formula or water from a bottle

Insufficient Glandular Development

Insufficient glandular development of the breast has been reported in a small number of

women and is an infrequent cause of inadequate milk supply. It is indicated by:
- The absence of typical breast changes during pregnancy
- No postpartum breast engorgement or lactogenesis
- Obvious abnormal development of at least one breast
- Inadequate milk production despite appropriate feeding routines and a good suckling stimulus

ADEQUATE MILK

If it appears that the infant is receiving an adequate amount of milk, the mother's concerns may be based on a lack of or inaccurate information or the infant may be experiencing a growth spurt.

Misinformation

Misinformation may be indicated by the mother's belief that:
- The infant is nursing too often
- The infant should follow the same feeding schedule as a bottle-fed baby
- Her breasts should feel as full as they did initially
- Her baby should sleep through the night
- She has been unable to hand-express or pump significant amounts of milk and assumes it indicates a lack of milk
- The infant's cries always indicate a need to be fed

Growth Spurt

A growth spurt is a period when the infant's demands for nursing increase (due to an increased caloric need, for growth) and the maternal supply lags behind this demand. This can occur any time during the first several months, although it is most common at three weeks, six weeks and three months of age.

Management

The most common response of women when they feel their milk supply is inadequate is to offer the infant a supplemental bottle. This usually worsens the problem by decreasing maternal milk production.

Misinformation

Many women feel their infant is nursing too often, not realizing that it is normal for young infants to nurse every one and one-half to three hours.

The mother should be reassured:
- That it is normal for a young infant to nurse every one and one-half to three hours
- That the feedings will be further apart as the baby gets older

Formula-fed babies usually eat less frequently than breastfed infants. This is due to the shorter digestion time for breast milk.

The mother should be counseled about the differences in breast- and bottle-fed babies' feeding patterns.

The mother's breast size normally decreases slightly after the initial postpartum period without any parallel decrease in breast milk production. The mother should be reassured that her breasts will eventually return to a more normal size while breastfeeding.

Newborn infants typically awaken every four to six hours during the night. It is unrealistic to expect an infant to sleep more than six hours at a time before the baby is eight to 12 weeks old. The mother should be counseled about normal infant sleeping patterns.

The baby's crying does not always indicate a need to be fed. The mother should be counseled on the management of an infant's crying (see Section #23).

It is difficult for many women to hand-express a significant quantity of milk beyond the initial postpartum period, as the infant is much more efficient at obtaining milk. The mother should be reassured that the baby is receiving adequate milk and that it is difficult to hand-express significant quantities of milk (see Section #2).

Growth Spurt

The mother should be questioned to determine her response to her infant's increased demand for milk and should be advised:

- To increase frequency of breastfeeding for three to four days
- To offer both breasts at each feeding. She may return to the first breast if the baby wants to continue nursing
- To discontinue the use of additional formula at this time if the infant is young
- That she will be able to meet the infant's needs by doing these things

Maternal Anxiety

Any situation causing stress and tension may produce maternal anxiety and may inhibit "let down." The mother should be counseled on the physiological need for additional rest during the initial breastfeeding period. The health care provider should suggest that the mother enlist the husband, friends or relatives to help with housework, cooking, the other children and other chores and that the mother take a warm bath before nursing and nurse in a quiet, partially darkened room away from distractions. She should be reassured that she is producing good quality milk.

Enlisting the support of influential "others" is critically important. In some instances, the health care provider may need to include the husband, friends or relatives in the counseling and advise them that breastfeeding is much more likely to be successful with their help.

Technique

In order to have an adequate milk supply, the mother must nurse frequently. The mother should:

- Understand the law of supply and demand. The more often she nurses, the more milk she will have if the infant is sucking appropriately
- Nurse the baby on demand every one and one-half to three hours
- Be sure baby is latched on correctly, with $3/4$ to 1 inch of areola in his mouth, and is suckling effectively
- Nurse the baby on both breasts at each feeding for at least 10 minutes on each breast

Maternal and Infant Diet

Maternal diet may affect the quantity and quality of breast milk. However, unless the mother is seriously malnourished, she will probably continue to produce sufficient quantities of breast milk, even if her diet is inadequate, though this will compromise her own nutritional status (see Section #6). The mother should drink six to eight glasses of fluid per day and consume 500 to 800 calories a day above the caloric intake recommended for non-lactating women.

Inappropriate feeding patterns of the infant may result in decreased milk supply. Under normal conditions, there is no need to provide supplemental water or formula before the baby is four to six weeks of age. These practices may result in "nipple confusion" or a satiated baby with no desire to nurse (see Sections #11, #12 and #25).

It may take four to six weeks to establish the mother's milk supply fully, after which time the supplemental formula or water may be introduced to the baby's diet if necessary. However, solid foods should not be introduced until the baby is developmentally ready (four to six months of age), since early introduction interferes with milk production and is not necessary to meet the infant's nutritional requirements (see Section #15).

Insufficient Glandular Development
When insufficient glandular development is diagnosed by a medical professional:
- The mother should be advised that the problem is not due to her breastfeeding performance
- The mother may continue to breastfeed; however, formula supplementation is necessary (see Section #11)

#17 Anxiety Regarding Quality of Breast Milk

Introduction

Early in their nursing experience, many women become overly concerned that their milk is "no good" or "not rich enough." These are often vague, undefined fears that are difficult to counteract. These feelings may arise from a lack of support for the mother's breastfeeding decision, misinformation regarding breastfeeding or concern for her infant's growth. When a woman voices these fears, it indicates her need for accurate information and supportive counseling. Without reassurance, many women who feel their milk is "no good" will discontinue nursing during the first few weeks.

Assessment

To provide appropriate counseling, the mother needs to be more specific about her concerns. The health care provider should determine the reason the mother feels her milk is "no good."

Most frequently, the causes of the mother's anxiety about the quality of her breast milk are due to:

- Lack of support
- Misinformation
- Concern about the infant's growth

Lack of support may be indicated by statements that imply:

- That her sister or mother couldn't breastfeed due to poor quality or insufficient milk supply

- That the infant's father is disinterested or antagonistic to her breastfeeding
- That she has few friends who have breast-fed
- That her physician or the health care providers seem disinterested in her nursing

Misinformation may be indicated by the mother's belief that:
- Her milk is too thin or watery
- The baby is allergic to her milk
- The baby is "refusing the breast"

Concern regarding inadequate infant growth may be indicated by the mother's belief that:
- The baby is not getting enough milk
- The baby is not gaining weight adequately
- Her milk does not satisfy the baby

Management
Support
Postpartum support is recognized as a critical factor in achieving a successful breastfeeding experience. The role of the "doula" or supportive individual is well-documented in other societies. The predominant mode of infant feeding in the United States and other developed countries remains commercial formulas. Therefore, many people may have had little exposure to breastfeeding. Unsuccessful breastfeeding experiences are usually related to inadequate support systems rather than poor quality milk.

The provider should:

- Refer the mother to local breastfeeding support groups, e.g., La Leche League or the Special Supplemental Nutrition Program for Women, Infants, and Children (WIC)
- Counsel the woman, instilling confidence in her mothering skills
- Enlist the involvement of the mother's support system (e.g., grandmothers, father, family and friends), emphasizing that the likelihood of a successful breastfeeding experience increases with their support (see Section #5)

Information

Many women feel that their milk is too thin, not realizing that breast milk normally is watery and blue. The fat content is low in the fore milk that the mother can see and higher in hind milk that she cannot see.

Few babies are truly allergic to breast milk. The mother should be counseled concerning the normal characteristics of breast milk and what the mother perceives as breast milk allergy. True breast milk allergy is rare.

The baby may be behaving in such a way that the mother feels he is refusing the breast because he does not like her milk or her milk is not good. He may not be latching on to the breast and sucking correctly because of poor suckling technique (see Section #25).

Growth

It is difficult for the mother to quantify the volume of breast milk her baby is ingesting. She should be reassured that the quantity of her milk is adequate if the baby is following a normal growth pattern.

It may take up to two weeks for a baby to regain its birth weight. Normal growth after this is $^1/_2$ to 1 ounce per day.

Many young babies normally have fussy periods that the mother may misinterpret as his not being satisfied or satiated with her breast milk (see Section #23).

The health care provider should:

- Offer the mother the opportunity to weigh her baby and document the growth
- Reassure the mother that the baby's weight gain is adequate
- Discuss normal fussy periods in young babies

#18 Sore Nipples

Introduction

When a woman states that she has breast pain, it is necessary to differentiate between sore nipples and other possible breast problems (see Section #19). Complaints of sore nipples are common during the first few weeks of nursing.

This problem is temporary and is most frequently caused by:

- Improper positioning of the infant
- Inadequate nursing schedule
- Improper nipple care

Nipple soreness usually begins on the second or third day after birth and is more pronounced at the beginning of the feeding.

Many women, not realizing that sore nipples are a temporary problem, may discontinue breastfeeding. It is important to encourage these women to continue nursing.

Assessment

In order to provide appropriate counseling to manage sore nipples, it is necessary to assess the cause of the problem. The mother should be questioned about potential problems in positioning, nursing schedule and nipple care or the use of a nipple shield. Sore nipples and cracked or bleeding nipples can also be caused by poor suckling (see Section #25) or a thrush infection (see Section #29).

Positioning

Improper positioning is indicated by nipple soreness only during the nursing session. Nipple soreness at times other than nursing usually indicates causes other than positioning.

Nursing Schedule

An inappropriate nursing schedule is indicated when the:

- Interval between nursing sessions is more than one and one-half to three hours
- Duration of nursing sessions is less than 10 minutes on each breast
- Baby is not nursing from both breasts at each feeding

Nipple Care

Improper nipple care is indicated when the mother is:

- Using soap or alcohol on her nipples
- Using a breast cream on her nipples that must be washed off
- Using a breast pad with a plastic liner
- Using a "bicycle horn"-type breast pump
- Using nipple shields

Management

For immediate relief of pain, the mother may place an ice cube on the nipple to numb it prior to nursing. She may also take acetaminophen 650 mg every four hours. Nipple soreness is usually caused by:

- Improper positioning
- Improper nursing schedule
- Improper nipple care

The mother should be advised to review proper nursing techniques to prevent further problems (see Section #10). Specific problems may be handled by suggesting that the mother follow the techniques offered below.

Improper Positioning

The mother may be holding the infant too far from the breast or the infant may not have the areola in his mouth completely. This improper infant positioning may cause the infant to chew on the nipple. The mother should be advised to:

- Position the baby correctly, with the baby facing the mother on his side and his arm around her waist
- After touching the baby's lips with the breast to elicit the rooting reflex and opening his mouth, pull the baby in close so he grasps $3/4$ to 1 inch of the areola in his mouth
- Change positions with each feeding to prevent pressure areas
- Touch the nipple directly to the baby's lips to encourage him to grasp the areola fully
- Break suction with her little finger before removing the baby from the breast

Nursing Schedule

Infrequent feeding may cause the infant to be so hungry that he will suck too vigorously, causing nipple pain. Infrequent feeding may also cause breast engorgement, which results in the baby's having difficulty manipulating the areola into his mouth. The infant then chews on the protruding nipple, causing discomfort. The mother should be advised:

- Not to discontinue nursing, even when nipples are cracked; sore nipples are only temporary
- To nurse the baby on demand at least every one and one-half to three hours
- To start each feeding on the least sore nipple

- To nurse for as long as the baby is hungry, at least 10 minutes on each breast
- Prior to nursing to soften the areola place warm cloths on the breasts and hand express some milk (see Section #2)
- To nurse from both breasts at each feeding

Improper Nipple Care

Improper nipple care is a frequent cause of sore nipples. There are numerous commercial products marketed that may actually harm the nipples. Soap and alcohol strip the natural oil from the nipple. Breast pads with plastic liners keep moisture on the nipples, exacerbating soreness. "Bicycle horn"-type pumps produce excessive negative pressure and are unsanitary. Nipple shields prevent the baby from attaching and sucking adequately.

Nipple care procedures should include instructions to the mother to:
- Air dry nipples after nursing
- Apply breast milk to the nipples, as it has healing properties itself
- Discontinue use of soap or alcohol and use plain water to clean the nipples
- Discontinue use of all breast creams that must be washed off
- Only use breast pads without plastic liners or use absorbent cloths such as terry cloth
- Discontinue use of "bicycle horn"-type breast pumps to express milk
- Use hand-expression, a cylindric manual pump or an electric pump to express milk
- Discontinue use of nipple shields

#19 Sore Breasts (Engorgement)

Introduction

When a woman indicates that she has breast pain, it is necessary to differentiate between engorgement, plugged ducts and mastitis. Other possible problems, such as sore nipples, may be indicated when the mother complains of sore breasts and should be differentiated and handled appropriately (see Section #18).

Sore breasts are usually caused by engorgement. Twelve to 48 hours postpartum, swelling of tissues and increased blood supply commonly cause tenderness. Later, engorgement from an oversupply of milk can occur whenever the baby has gone longer than usual without nursing.

When the mother complains of sore breasts, it is important to be certain that there are no signs of infection, such as:

- Fever
- Malaise
- Redness
- Localized tenderness

Infection usually occurs when the breasts have been inadequately emptied for an extended period; therefore, frequent nursing will help prevent infection. If infection in the breast (mastitis) does occur, it must be treated with antibiotics. The mother does not need to discontinue nursing because of infection.

Assessment

In order to provide appropriate counseling to manage sore breasts, it is important to differentiate between engorgement, plugged ducts and mastitis. These may co-exist and in some cases form a continuum.

Engorgement
Engorgement is indicated by:
- Full, hard, tender breasts
- No localized tenderness or lumps
- No signs of mastitis
- Recent history of infrequent or short nursing periods
- Occurrence commonly at two to five days postpartum

Plugged Milk Ducts
Plugged milk ducts are indicated by:
- Localized tender spot on the breast
- Palpable lump in the breast
- No signs of mastitis

Mastitis
Mastitis is indicated by:
- Localized or generalized redness and extreme tenderness of the breast
- Fever and/or chills
- Malaise and fatigue
- Recent history of plugged ducts

Management
The most important management technique for all of these conditions is for the mother to continue nursing on both the affected and unaffected breasts. In most instances, this problem can be prevented by frequent, on-demand, adequate nursing sessions.

Engorgement

Unrelieved engorgement will rapidly result in involution of mammary glandular tissue, causing decreased milk production. It can also inhibit let-down if the baby is unable to latch on correctly, with enough of the areola in his mouth. Engorgement must be treated primarily by emptying the breasts. The mother should be advised to:

- Nurse frequently
- Hand-express some milk prior to nursing to soften the breast and after nursing to remove excess milk (see Section #2)
- Nurse in different positions, e.g., sitting up, lying down (see Section #10)
- Take a hot shower or apply warm compresses to the breasts prior to nursing
- Nurse during the night, waking the baby if necessary
- Restrict the use of supplemental water or formula (see Sections #11 and #12)
- Wear a good support bra with non-elastic straps that do not constrict soft tissue in the axilla

Plugged Ducts

The mother should be counseled to:

- Nurse frequently from both breasts
- Get plenty of rest
- Nurse in different positions
- Nurse during the night
- Apply warm compresses to the affected area
- Massage the breast gently from the affected area down toward the nipple

- Contact her physician if the lump does not resolve itself within one week
- Know the signs of mastitis and be aware that she should contact her physician if it develops

Mastitis

The mother should be counseled to:
- Nurse frequently
- Apply warm compresses to affected areas
- Contact her physician for antibiotic treatment (see Section #20)
- Rest in bed as much as possible

Prevention

Engorgement, plugged ducts and mastitis are usually preventable through:
- Frequent nursing
- Nursing on demand every one and one-half to three hours
- Nursing from both breasts at each feeding
- Avoiding prolonged time between nursing sessions (nighttime or physical separations)
- Avoiding tight or restrictive bras

#20 Mastitis

Introduction

Mastitis is an infection in the breast tissue, usually preceded by:
- Nipple abrasion
- An obstructed duct
- Engorgement

Infection usually occurs when the breasts have been inadequately emptied for an extended period of time. Therefore, frequent nursing will help prevent mastitis.

The highest incidence of mastitis occurs in the second or third week postpartum. A poorly nourished, fatigued woman is more susceptible to infection. There is some indication that mastitis is more common among working women. If the infection does occur, the mother must be treated with antibiotics and rest, but does not need to discontinue nursing. In fact, it is necessary for the mother to empty the breast frequently.

Assessment

When a women indicates that she has breast pain, it is necessary to differentiate between engorgement, plugged ducts and mastitis (see Section #19).

Mastitis is indicated by:
- Localized or generalized redness or extreme tenderness of the breast
- Fever and/or chills
- Malaise and fatigue

Management

Mastitis must be treated until all signs of infection are gone. If not, the likelihood of recurrence increases and may lead to more serious complications such as sepsis or breast abscesses.

If infection is present, the mother must be encouraged to continue nursing and the infection must be treated with antibiotics. A suggested course of antibiotic treatment may be one of the following:

- Ampicillin 500 mg four times per day for 10 days
- Erythromycin 500 mg four times per day for two days, followed by 250 mg four times per day for eight days
- Dicloxacillin 250 mg four times per day for 10 days
- Mild analgesics (e.g., acetaminophen)

20.

Additionally, it is necessary to empty the infected breast even if it requires manual expressing or pumping.

The mother should be counseled to:

- Continue nursing
- Nurse frequently
- Apply warm compresses or ice packs to affected area
- Rest as much as possible; bed rest is extremely important
- Offer the baby the infected breast first
- Drink plenty of fluids
- Take analgesics for pain
- Wear an appropriately fitting bra (one that is not too tight)

#21 Leaking Breasts

Introduction

Milk leaking from the breasts is normal and will help relieve engorgement in the early weeks. It seems to be more common in first-time mothers. It may last anywhere from a few days to several months but tends to occur more frequently in the first few weeks. Common stimuli causing leakage include:

- Full breasts
- A crying infant
- Sexual intercourse

Management

There is no way to prevent normal leakage of milk. One means of managing it is to help the mother deal with the leakage to avoid socially awkward situations.

The mother should be advised that:

- Frequent nursing will empty the breasts and reduce the likelihood of leakage
- She may use nursing pads or other absorbable material in her bra to absorb leakage
- She should not use plastic-lined nursing pads
- She may temporarily reduce leakage by briefly pressing the palm of her hand on the leaking breast
- She may wear a loose sweater or a jacket to cover up leaks on her clothes
- Leakage during sexual intercourse or orgasm is normal and not harmful in any way
- Nursing prior to sexual intercourse will empty the breasts and help eliminate the leakage
- Leakage is only temporary

NOTES

21.

#22 Maternal Illness

Introduction

There are very few maternal illnesses that are contraindications to breastfeeding. Mothers sometimes feel that they should not nurse their babies if they themselves are sick. However, by the time the illness has manifested itself, an infant has been exposed and will continue to be exposed to the mother even if he is bottle-fed.

Breastfeeding continues to provide protection to the baby because of the anti-infective properties of breast milk (see Section #1).

Assessment

It should first be determined if the mother is under the care of a physician for any serious illness or condition. A limited number of serious illnesses may preclude breastfeeding.

Secondly, it should be determined if the mother is on medications that may affect the breast milk (see Section #7).

Thirdly, it should be determined if the mother has a common illness such as:

- An upper respiratory infection
- Gastroenteritis
- Urinary tract infection
- Flu

These common illnesses do not preclude breastfeeding.

Management

Under most circumstances, a woman does not need to discontinue nursing because she is ill. However, there are a limited number of illnesses that are contraindications to breastfeeding. These include:

- Active tuberculosis
- HIV infections/AIDS
- Alcoholism
- Heroin addiction
- Malaria
- Severe chronic disease resulting in maternal malnourishment

Breastfeeding by women with cystic fibrosis is possible, as the milk secreted by these women appears to be physiologically normal. Such women require special management, and the nutritional status of both the mother and infant must be carefully monitored.

Hepatitis B carrier mothers may breastfeed if the infant has received appropriate hepatitis B prophylaxis with HBIG and HB vaccine.

There are also a few other maternal illnesses for which the medications prescribed may be contraindicated for breastfeeding (see Section #7).

22.

#23 Fussy Infant

Introduction

Newborns and young infants frequently have fussy periods. Mothers often erroneously feel that their milk causes the fussiness, and that may prompt them to wean the baby prematurely. This complaint may be brought to the attention of the health care provider most frequently by first-time mothers who may have unrealistic expectations for their young infants.

Times when babies are normally fussy include:

- The first few days at home when the baby is going through a normal adjustment period
- Following periods of excessive external stimulation (e.g., large family gatherings)
- In the late afternoons and early evenings, usually between 4 and 11 p.m. daily

Other less common causes of fussiness include:

- Illness in the infant
- Poor nursing technique
- Maternal anxiety
- Maternal diet

Assessment

Illness

The health care provider should determine if the baby has diarrhea, fever or other signs of illness.

Poor Nursing Technique

Poor nursing technique may result in inadequate caloric intake by the infant and fussy behavior. Poor nursing technique is indicated when:

- The interval between nursing sessions is more than one and one-half to three hours
- The duration of nursing sessions is less than 10 minutes on each breast
- The mother is not nursing from both breasts at each feeding
- The mother is not burping the baby adequately during and after feedings
- There is inappropriate use of rubber nipples, causing "nipple confusion" (see Section #25)
- There is poor positioning of the infant (see Section #10)
- The baby is not grasping the areola and sucking effectively (see Section #10)

Maternal Anxiety

The infant of an anxious mother will mirror the mother's anxiety and may be unusually fussy.

Maternal anxiety is indicated by:

- Statements that suggest a lack of confidence in her caretaking abilities
- Evidence that suggests she is in a stressful environment
- History of inadequate rest, resulting in fatigue
- The mother's worry that the baby does not like her breast milk (see Section #17)
- The mother's worry that the baby is not getting enough breast milk (see Section #16)
- Lack of maternal support network, e.g., the mother does not have many friends, the grandmother is unavailable, the mother's partner or husband is disinterested or otherwise uninvolved in the breastfeeding situation

Maternal Diet

Occasionally certain foods the mother consumes, particularly some fruits and vegetables, may cause fussiness in the infant. However, it may be quite difficult to determine the offending food accurately (with the exception of caffeine-containing substances, e.g., coffee, cola drinks, etc.) This uncertainty may be frustrating to the mother. If a woman suspects a particular food is causing fussiness, she should observe the infant for a 24-hour period after consumption of that food to assess its effect on the infant. However, it may be difficult for the mother to sort out the effect of the food from everything else to which the infant is exposed; additionally, it may be that any effect of the food on the infant will not be evident within a 24-hour period (see Section #6). Attention to other potential causes of infant fussiness may prove to be more productive.

Management

A fussy infant does not indicate a need to discontinue breastfeeding. To prevent mothers from discontinuing breastfeeding, the health care provider should counsel the mother about:

- Normal infant behavior
- Illness in the infant
- Proper nursing techniques
- Maternal anxiety
- Maternal diet

Normal Infant Behavior

The mother may simply be too anxious. She may need reassurance or information. She should be informed that:

- The baby's behavior is normal
- Babies are typically fussy the first few days at home, following periods of excessive stimulation and in the late afternoon and evenings
- Most infants outgrow fussiness by three months of age
- The baby may be more hungry during the evening hours and can appropriately be nursed every one to one and one-half hours at this time
- She should try to arrange for breaks from the infant, particularly after lactation is established
- Carrying the infant when he is not crying should increase the amount of satisfied awake time. A front pack or pouch works well for this, as the infant can have eye contact with the mother, can hear the mother's heartbeat and can enjoy the mother's softness
- Comforting techniques for infants include holding, rocking, walking or swaddling. Slow rhythmic motions, such as infant swings or car rides, often quiet fussy babies
- Very young babies will not be spoiled by holding them; babies need to be held, loved and talked to
- If the baby's diapers are dry and the mother has fed, burped and held the fussy baby, it is appropriate to put him to bed and let him cry awhile

Illness

If the infant shows signs of illness, appropriate medical management is necessary.

Nursing Techniques

The health care provider should observe a feeding to determine if appropriate techniques are being used (see Section #10) and advise the mother that:

- The interval between nursing sessions should not usually be less than one and one-half hours or more than three hours
- She should not limit the length of the feedings; the baby should nurse as long as he desires
- She should nurse from both breasts at each feeding
- She should discontinue use of rubber nipples
- The baby needs to grasp the areola fully and suck effectively
- If the mother's breasts are engorged, she should hand-express milk to soften the breast (see Section #2)

Maternal Anxiety

The health care provider should reassure the mother that she is doing a good job. Promoting the development of parental confidence is very important. A relaxed mother means a relaxed baby.

Relaxation techniques also should be discussed with the mother. Suggestions for relaxation may include:

- A warm shower or bath
- A quiet environment
- A warm drink

The provider should advise the mother to ask for help, if possible, from relatives or friends to give the mother time to relax and regain her energies. Others should be brought in to the caretaking process. The physician or lactation consultant may need to talk to the father or other individuals to enlist their support. It is clear that a woman will have a difficult time nursing successfully without support of family and/or friends, even with assistance from a health care provider. If no support help is available, the mother should try to take her own needs into account. She should let the housework go and nap when the baby is sleeping. If appropriate, the mother may be referred to a mental health care provider.

Maternal Diet

The mother should discontinue ingesting specific foods if it is clear that they are related to the baby's fussiness. Ingestion of caffeine-containing substances should cease immediately. The provider should ensure the nutritional adequacy of the mother's diet by suggesting alternatives for the eliminated foods, if necessary. If the baby's fussiness does not abate, the mother may reintroduce the suspected foods into her diet and consider other possible causes of fussiness.

#24 Sleepy Infant

Introduction

Some young infants are "sleepy babies." These infants sleep longer than normal intervals and may be so undemanding that adequate nursing is not established. This problem manifests itself through:

- Unsuccessful nippling
- Infrequent nursing sessions
- Poor weight gain

Assessment

A "sleepy baby" can be detected in various ways but must be differentiated from an infant who is lethargic because of illness. A "sleepy baby" may be indicated by:

- Improper attachment to the nipple when breastfeeding (see Section #10)
- An infant who sleeps more than four hours at a time
- An infant who appears to be uninterested in nursing and falls asleep at the breast
- An infant who shows poor weight gain
- The mother's reports that her milk is "no good" (see Section #17)

Management

If the baby has other signs of illness or jaundice, appropriate medical management is necessary.

If the baby is sleepy and has nippling or nursing difficulty, he should be awakened for nursing at least every three to four hours.

The mother should be advised to:

- Unwrap the infant from blankets and stimulate him by:
  - Rubbing his back or feet
  - Talking to him
  - Trying to establish eye-to-eye contact
  - Sitting him in her lap with his chin in her hand
- Understand:
  - Correct nursing positions
  - The rooting reflex
  - How to attach the baby to the breast (see Section #10)
  - How to express milk into the baby's mouth to whet his appetite
- Handle the baby by:
  - Changing diapers before nursing
  - Applying lotion to baby's arms and legs
  - Giving a gentle rub-down for five to 10 minutes
  - Burping the baby
- Avoid giving the baby a bottle, as this can cause "nipple confusion" and make the baby too full to nurse (see Section #25)
- Express milk to avoid engorgement and interruption of milk supply, if the baby is not nursing successfully

24.

#25 Breast Refusal (Poor Suckling)

Introduction

Sometimes a mother will report that her baby is "refusing the breast." The baby does not latch on and suck effectively. He just chews on the nipple or he pushes the nipple out of his mouth. He throws back his head, arches his back and cries. The mother may think her milk is "no good" or that the baby does not like it. She may feel rejected and frustrated. This behavior may actually indicate that the baby is not sucking correctly.

Another mother may report that baby "nurses all the time" but that he is not gaining weight adequately and has poor urinary output indicating he is not getting enough milk. This may also be a clue to incorrect sucking.

Poor suckling can be caused by the baby being positioned incorrectly so that he does not get enough of the areola in his mouth to enable him to draw out the milk or to trigger the letdown reflex. It can be caused by "negative" or "flutter" sucking, which means the baby is using his tongue incorrectly. Poor suckling can be caused by nipple confusion when the baby has been given rubber nipples.

Failure to suck effectively, for any reason, may result in:

- Decreased milk supply
- Frustration with nursing by both mother and infant
- Abandonment of breastfeeding

Assessment

Poor sucking can be caused by:

- Improper positioning of the infant on the breast
- Negative or flutter sucking
- Nipple confusion

In order to assess the baby's suckling behavior accurately, it is necessary to:

- Observe the baby nursing at the breast
- Notice the sounds of the infant's swallowing and the motion of the masseter (jaw muscle)
- Check the baby's tongue position and sucking technique with your finger
- Obtain a history on the use of rubber nipples, pacifiers or nipple shields

Improper Positioning

Proper positioning begins at the first feeding. It is important to put the infant to the breast as soon after birth as possible. However, it is best not to force the infant onto the breast if he is not exhibiting the rooting reflex. Infants should not be forced to nurse, particularly when crying.

25.

Improper positioning may be identified while observing a nursing session. It is indicated when:

- The baby has an insufficient amount of the areola in his mouth (less than $3/4$ to 1 inch)
- The baby is chewing on the protruding nipple
- The baby has his lower lip folded in so he is sucking it, obstructing access to the nipple
- The mother complains of sore, cracked or bleeding nipples (see Section #18)

Negative or Flutter Sucking

To check the baby's suck with her finger the mother should:

- Stroke the baby's cheeks and lips to elicit the rooting reflex
- When the baby opens his mouth, slip her index or fifth finger with the finger pad facing upward into the mouth and gently rub the baby's soft palate

Incorrect sucking action (negative or flutter sucking) is indicated when:

- The baby's tongue is on the roof of his mouth, pushing against the nipple
- The back of the baby's tongue is pulled up, causing the baby to gag when the nipple or a finger is inserted into his mouth
- The wavelike motion of the tongue is reversed, moving from back to front

Correct tongue positioning and sucking is indicated when:

- The tongue lies under the nipple with the tip extended forward to the lips and with the sides curling around and grasping the nipple
- The sucking motion starts at the tip and ripples back, causing suction both upwards against the nipple and back towards the throat

Nipple Confusion

The term "nipple confusion" refers to an infant who is unable to grasp or who has difficulty grasping the mother's soft nipple. This generally develops in young infants who have been exposed to artificial nipples and/or pacifiers. Sucking rubber nipples requires a different tongue action than sucking the mother's nipple, and it is easier for the infant to get milk from a bottle than from the breast.

Nipple confusion is indicated when the baby:
- Has been offered rubber nipples early
- Seems to refuse the breast but feeds well from the bottle
- Suckles incorrectly and ineffectively at the breast

Management
Positioning

In order to suck effectively, the baby must have approximately $3/4$ to 1 inch of the areola drawn into his mouth.

The mother should be advised:
- To position the baby correctly at the breast (see Section #10)
- To stroke the area around the baby's mouth and touch his lips with the nipple to elicit the rooting reflex
- To draw the baby in quickly as soon as his mouth is open so he can grasp the areola fully
- That if the baby clamps his mouth closed too quickly or does not open his mouth wide enough, the mother may need to hold his mouth open by putting pressure on his chin with her finger until the baby has a firm grasp of the areola and enough suction to maintain the correct position

Negative or Flutter Sucking

The baby needs to be trained to suck correctly and effectively. In order to do this, the mother needs to understand proper sucking technique.

She should be counseled regarding the proper sucking technique and training of the infant. To train the baby to suck correctly the mother should:

- With the index finger, stroke the baby's cheeks and lips and massage his gums
- Insert the finger with the pad up against the palate, gently rubbing the hard palate back towards the soft palate
- When the baby starts to suck, press the finger down and forward against the tongue, allowing the baby to suck against the pressure of the back of the finger
- Alternate rubbing the palate with the finger pad and exerting pressure on the tongue
- Follow this procedure before each feeding, during the feeding if necessary and when the baby needs pacifying, until he learns the proper technique; this may take one to two weeks
- Give the baby expressed breast milk with a dropper, cup or spoon or Lact-Aid until he learns to suck effectively at the breast
- Not introduce a rubber nipple throughout this training

Nipple Confusion

An infant with poor suckling can usually still get the easily obtainable milk from a bottle with a rubber nipple. Giving him a rubber nipple reinforces poor sucking and makes it harder for him to learn to suckle at the breast. Being offered two kinds of nipples when his suck is already poor causes the baby to be confused and frustrated.

It is best to prevent this confusion by not offering any rubber nipples until breastfeeding is fully established.

If the baby is taking a bottle but refusing the breast the mother should:

- Discontinue use of artificial nipples, including pacifiers and nipple shields
- Position the infant properly as outlined in *Positioning*
- Offer the breast often
- Offer the breast when the baby is responsive but not excessively hungry
- Drip breast milk onto the nipple to entice the infant to suck at the beginning of each feeding
- Initiate training to enable the baby to suck correctly as outlined in *Negative or Flutter Sucking*
- Be advised that breast shields worn between feedings, use of manual or pump expression prior to nursing and rolling the nipple between thumb and forefinger may enhance nipple protractility and make it easier for the infant to grasp
- Give the baby expressed breast milk with a dropper, cup or spoon or Lact-Aid until he learns to suck effectively
- Be advised that, to maintain her milk supply, she may empty her breasts after each feeding by hand-expression or use of a pump

Poor suckling is a particularly difficult problem for both mother and baby. At a time when she is tired and emotionally labile herself, the mother must be patient with a fussy, often hungry infant while he learns to nurse effectively. She needs as much support as can be given by the health care provider or counselor and by the family.

#26 Infant Diarrhea

Introduction

Stools of a newborn breastfed infant are frequent and watery, causing some mothers to believe that the baby has diarrhea. A normally active gastrocolic reflex can result in a bowel movement following nearly every feeding. Often the report of diarrhea in the breastfed infant represents a normal stooling pattern. However, when it truly exists, diarrhea can be a serious problem for infants and must be identified and treated.

Assessment

In order to provide appropriate counseling to manage this problem, it is necessary to determine the presence or absence of illness or dehydration as well as the stool frequency and consistency.

Normal breastfed infant's stools:
- Are frequent and usually follow each feeding
- May occur every two hours
- Are often runny and watery
- May be greenish to yellow-orange in color; in the absence of other signs of illness, this is normal

Signs and symptoms of illness or dehydration may include:
- Blood or mucus in stool
- Fever
- Dry mouth and tongue
- A sunken fontanel
- Rapid breathing
- Four or fewer wet diapers within 24 hours
- Refusal of the infant to feed

Management

If the baby has no sign of illness, the mother should be counseled regarding the normal stooling pattern of breastfed infants and reassured that the infant does not have diarrhea.

If signs and symptoms of illness are present, the infant should receive appropriate hydration and be referred for medical management.

26.

#27 Infant Constipation

Introduction

Constipation is defined as hard dry stools and does not relate to the frequency of stooling or to grunting with stooling. Constipation is very unusual in breastfed babies.

Many infants, especially at three to four months of age, pass stools infrequently. It is normal for some breastfed infants to stool as infrequently as every seven to 10 days.

Assessment

It is necessary to differentiate the rare infant who truly is constipated from the normal infant whose mother reports that he is constipated. The frequency and consistency of stools must be noted to determine true constipation.

Mothers commonly mistake the following infant behavior for constipation:
- Infant's grunting or making noises when stooling
- Grimacing when passing stools
- Infrequent stools that are of normal consistency

Signs of true constipation are stools that are:
- Dry
- Hard
- Infrequent

Constipation probably indicates that other foods have been added to the infant's diet or that the infant is ill.

Management

The mother who reports constipation in her breastfed infant usually needs education and counseling. The mother needs to be reassured and to be informed that:

- Constipation refers to hard, dry stools, not the frequency of stooling
- Babies may stool as seldom as every seven to 10 days and still not be constipated if stools are soft
- The baby's grunting and making grimaces is probably not a sign of constipation
- She should not give laxatives or use suppositories

If the infant is truly constipated, the mother should be questioned as to whether formula, milk or solid foods have been introduced into the infant's diet. If these are inappropriate, she should be advised to discontinue use of these supplemental foods (see Section #15).

27.

#28 Jaundice

Introduction

Jaundice in the newborn is a common problem. During the 1960s the concept of "breast milk jaundice" became established to explain the observation that occasionally breastfed infants experienced prolonged jaundice with peaks in bilirubin levels during the second week. It is now generally accepted that bilirubin levels in "physiologic jaundice" peak at 72 hours and diminish thereafter.

The natural history of jaundice in breastfed infants is a matter of some controversy. However, recent studies have demonstrated that after the fourth postpartum day, a larger proportion of breastfed infants maintain elevated bilirubin levels that may last for up to three weeks. Many authorities now feel that breastfeeding jaundice can occur as early as the third or fourth day of life and that up to 20 percent of breastfed infants will have peak bilirubin concentrations greater than 12 mg/dl. Jaundice and breastfeeding are clearly associated, and often breastfeeding is the only apparent cause for hyperbilirubinemia.

Two separate patterns must be considered when investigating the breastfed infant with jaundice. The more common early onset pattern has peak bilirubin levels at four to five days of age. The infrequent late onset pattern has peak bilirubin levels at two weeks of age. The etiologies of these two conditions are probably different, with the early onset type related to inadequate milk intake and infrequency of feedings and the late onset type related to factors in the milk that inhibit bilirubin conjugation and excretion.

Assessment

Many breastfed infants may develop jaundice with peak bilirubin levels above the established range accepted for physiologic jaundice.

Breastfeeding, as the cause of hyper-bilirubinemia, should be strongly considered and investigated prior to extensive investigations for other causes. The healthy breastfeeding infant with indirect hyperbilirubinemia, a normal direct bilirubin level and normal findings (other than jaundice) on physical examination may be presumed to have breastfeeding-related jaundice and may not require further laboratory investigation.

Management

The management of breastfeeding-related jaundice usually consists of monitoring the infant's bilirubin status and reassurance to the mother. Although temporary interruption of breastfeeding with a consequent reduction in bilirubin concentration may serve as a useful diagnostic tool, it is almost never necessary since bilirubin levels seldom reach significant concentrations at or near the risk level for toxicity. Bilirubin encephalopathy has never been reported in relation to breast-feeding, and bilirubin concentrations below 17-18 mg/dl may be considered safe in full-term, otherwise healthy infants. Increasingly, management of breastfeeding-related jaundice excludes discontinuation of breastfeeding.

28.

Early Onset Jaundice

The most effective management of early onset breastfeeding jaundice is prevention. The clinician must support the breastfeeding mother to ensure that the infant begins nursing as soon following the delivery as possible and that he nurses successfully at frequent intervals. Mothers should be encouraged to nurse infants frequently on demand every one and one-half to three hours, and water supplementation should be avoided as it has no effect on bilirubin concentration. Mild to moderate hyperbilirubinemia (total bilirubin less than 15 mg/dl) will usually be self-limited and require no treatment.

Early onset breastfeeding jaundice may be managed by:

- Monitoring serum bilirubin levels on an out-patient basis
- If significant hyperbilirubinemia develops (concentrations approaching 15 to 16 mg/dl in full-term, health infants), temporarily discontinuing breastfeeding for 24 to 48 hours may be considered
- Supplementing breastfeeding with formula
- Counseling the mother to maintain lactation by expressing breast milk during this interruption of nursing (see Section #2)
- Resuming breastfeeding after a significant decrease in bilirubin levels confirms the diagnosis (a decrease of at least 2 mg/dl)

Breastfeeding support, both in-hospital and post-discharge, should be provided to all mothers of newborn infants. Mothers especially likely to benefit from organized support services are those having infants with jaundice, since these mothers are more likely to discontinue breastfeeding in the first month than are mothers of infants without such complications.

Late Onset Jaundice

Many infants with late onset jaundice will develop only mild to moderate hyperbilirubinemia. After eliminating the major treatable causes of prolonged unconjugated hyperbilirubinemia, these infants may be monitored without specific treatment until the condition spontaneously resolves, usually during the second month. The rare infant with late onset breastfeeding jaundice associated with hyperbilirubinemia in the range of 19 to 20 mg/dl may be managed by:

- Discontinuing breastfeeding for a period of 24 to 48 hours
- Establishing diagnosis by documenting at least a 2 mg/dl decrease in the level of serum bilirubin
- Supplementing breastfeeding with formula
- Counseling the mother to maintain lactation by expressing breast milk during this interruption of nursing
- Resuming breastfeeding after a significant decrease in bilirubin levels confirms the diagnosis
- Monitoring bilirubin levels, which should demonstrate a slow but steady decrease

Phototherapy

Phototherapy is not generally indicated in the treatment of breastfeeding-related jaundice, which can almost always be managed on an outpatient basis. Some authorities recommend phototherapy if the bilirubin level exceeds 17 mg/dl. However, the majority of infants with these levels can be successfully managed with temporary discontinuance of breastfeeding alone. If bilirubin levels do not decrease significantly after temporary discontinuance of breastfeeding, breast milk is probably not the cause. Breastfeeding should be resumed and other possible etiologies investigated.

NOTES

#29 Thrush

Introduction

Thrush is a common fungal infection of the oral mucosa in young infants. The infection may spread to the mother's nipples, causing soreness (see Section #18).

Assessment

Thrush can be diagnosed by the presence of white plaque on the infant's oral mucosa and tongue. This may cause poor nippling or a superficial skin infection on the mother's nipples. Maternal complaints of severe pain and nipple/breast redness is evidence of thrush even in the absence of white patches in the baby's mouth. The presence of thrush should be considered when the mother complains of sore nipples.

Management

Both the mother and baby must be treated simultaneously even if only one shows evidence of thrush. If both are not treated, continuous reinfection occurs and chronic thrush results.

The infant's infection should be treated with Nystatin oral suspension one ml in each side of the mouth three times per day after feeding until resolved.

The mother's infection should be treated with Nystatin ointment applied to the nipple three times per day after feeding until resolved.

The mother should be counseled to continue nursing since the infection will clear promptly when properly treated.

NOTES

29

#30 Breast Preference

Introduction

Some babies seem to prefer one breast and consistently refuse to nurse from the other. There is usually no apparent reason for this preference. Perhaps the mother holds the baby more comfortably and is more relaxed holding the baby in one arm than the other. Perhaps the baby prefers to lie on one side rather than the other.

This preference is usually shown during the first week or two and lasts only a short while. However, it is upsetting to a new mother who does not know what to do about the baby's refusal of one breast, and she often fears the baby will not get enough milk from just one breast.

Management

Often a change in nursing position or other nursing technique will be helpful in managing breast preference. In addition, the mother should be advised to:

- Move the baby from the preferred breast to the other without turning him; he is then being held in the "football hold" on the other side
- Offer the rejected breast first, when baby is most hungry
- Nurse the baby when he is sleepy and less aware
- Pump milk from the rejected breast to maintain milk supply and prevent engorgement in that breast
- Darken the room to reduce the baby's visual orientation

The mother should be reassured that:
- The baby's preference will probably pass in a few days
- Even in the rare case when the baby continues to take only one breast, the milk supply in that breast will be adequate to feed the baby and supplemental formula is not necessary

30.

References

1. Aberman S, Kirchhoff KT: Infant-feeding practice: Mothers' decision making. JOGN Nurs Sept/Oct 1985;394-398.

2. Adams JA, Hey DJ, Hall RT: Incidence of hyperbilirubinemia in breast- vs. formula-fed infants. Clin Ped 1985;24(2):69-73.

3. Agre F: The relationship of mode of infant feeding and location of care to frequency of infection. Am J Dis Child 1985;139:809-811.

4. Alberti KGMM: Preventing insulin dependent diabetes mellitus (letter). BMJ 1993; 307:1435-1436.

5. Allen LH, Pelto GH: Research on determinants of breastfeeding duration: Suggestions for biocultural studies. Med Anthro 1985;Spring:97-105.

6. American Academy of Pediatrics: The promotion of breastfeeding. Pediatrics 1982; 69:654-661.

7. American Academy of Pediatrics, Committee on Drugs: Breastfeeding and contraception. Pediatrics 1981;68(1):138-140.

8. American Academy of Pediatrics, Committee on Nutrition: Nutrition and lactation. Pediatrics 1981;68(3):435-443.

9. American Dietetic Association. Position of the ADA: Promotion of breastfeeding. J Am Diet Assoc 1986;86(11):1580-1585.

10. American Public Health Association Resolution 8226: Breastfeeding. Adopted 1982.

11. Anderson L, Parker R: Day care center attendance and hospitalization for lower respiratory tract illness. Pediatrics 1988; 82(3):300-308.

12. Anholm P, Hancock C: Breastfeeding: A preventive approach to health care in infancy. Issues Compr Pediatr Nurs 1986;9:1-10.

13. Arafat I, Allen DE, Fox JE: Maternal practice and attitudes toward breastfeeding. JOGN Nurs March/April 1981;91-95.

14. Arango JO: Promoting breastfeeding: A national perspective. Public Health Reports 1984;99(6):559-565.

15. Astarita C, Harris R: An epidemiological study of atopy in children. Clin Allergy 1988;18(4):341-350.

16. Athex DJ: Breastfeeding and atopic eczema. Brit Med J 1983;287(6395):775-776.

17. Auerbach KG: Employed breastfeeding mothers: Problems they encounter. Birth 1984;11:1720.

18. Auerbach KG: The effect of nipple shields on maternal milk volume. JOGN Nurs 1990; 19(5):419-427.

19. Auerbach KG: The influence of lactation consultant contact on breastfeeding duration in a low-income population. Nebr Med J 1985;Sept:341-346.

20. Auerbach KG: Nipple confusion (letter). Pediatrics 1993;92(2):299-300.

21. Auerbach KG, Gartner LM: Breastfeeding and human milk: Their association with jaundice in the neonate. J Am Med Women's Assoc 1987;40:89-107.

22. Auerbach KG, Guss E: Health care workers who breastfeed: Implications for patient management. JOGN Nurs 1985;July/Aug: 111-115.

23. Avila H, Arroyo P, Garcia D et al: Factors determining the suspension of breastfeeding in an urban population group. Bull Pan Am Hlth Organ 1980;14(3):286-292.

24. Avoa A, Fischer PR: The influence of perinatal instruction about breastfeeding on neonatal weight loss. Pediatrics 1990;86(2):313-314.

25. Axelson ML, Kurinij N, Sahlroot JT: Primiparas' beliefs about breastfeeding. J Am Diet Assoc 1985;85(1):77-79.

26. Baisch M, Fox R: Breastfeeding attitudes and practices among adolescents. J Adolesc Hlth Care 1989:10(1):41-45.

27. Ballard P: Breastfeeding for the working mother. Issues Compr Pediatr Nurs 1983; 6:249-259.

28. Baranowski T, Bee DE, Rassin DK et al: Social support, social influence, ethnicity and the breastfeeding decision. Soc Sci Med 1983;17(21):1599-1611.

29. Barber-Madden R, Cowell C, Petschek MA, Glanz K: Nutrition for pregnant and lactating women: Implications for worksite health promotion. J Nutr Educ 1986;18(1):S72-S75.

30. Bauchner H, Leventhal JM, Shapiro ED: Studies of breastfeeding and infections: How good is the evidence? JAMA 1986;256(7):887-892.

31. Bergevin YU, Dougherty C, Kramer MS: Do infant formula samples shorten the duration of breastfeeding? Lancet 1983;1148-1151.

32. Bernard-Bonnin A, Statchenko S: Hospital practices and breastfeeding duration: A meta-analysis of controlled trials. Birth 1989; 16(2):64-66.

33. Bevan ML, Mosley D, Lobach KS, Solimano GR: Factors influencing breastfeeding in an urban WIC program. J Am Diet Assoc 1984;84(1):563-567.

34. Bhaskaram P, Hemalatha P, Islam A: Zinc status in breastfed infants (letter): Lancet 1992;340:1416-1417.

35. Bhowmick SK, Johnson KR, Rettig KR: Rickets caused by vitamin D deficiency in breastfed infants in the southern United States (letter). AJDC 1991; 145:127-130.

36. Biegelson D, Cowell C, Goldberg D: Breastfeeding practices in a low-income population in New York City: A study of selected health department child health stations. JADA 1986;86(1):90-91.

37. Borch-Johnsen K, Mandrup-Poulsen T, Zachau-Christiansen B et al: Relation between breastfeeding and incidence rates of insulin-dependent diabetes mellitus. Lancet 1984:1083-1086.

38. Borovies DL: Assessing and managing pain in breastfeeding mothers. MCN 1984;9:272-276.

39. Breastfeeding and Human Lactation, Report of the Surgeon General's Workshop. U.S. Department of Health and Human Services, Public Health Service, Health Resources and Services Administration, 1984.

40. Breastfeeding prevents otitis media. Nutr Rev 1983;41:241-242.

41. Brodie MJ: Drugs and breastfeeding. The Practitioner 1986;230:483-485.

42. Brooten D, Brown L, Hollingsworth A et al: Breast milk jaundice. JOGN Nurs 1983:May/June:220-223.

43. Bryant CA: The impact of kin, friend, and neighbor networks on infant feeding practices. 1982;16:1757-1765.

44. Burr ML: Does infant feeding affect the risk of allergy? Arch Dis Child 1983;58:561-565.

45. Butte NF, Wong WW, Ferlic L et al: Energy expenditure and deposition of breastfed and formula fed infants during early infancy. Pediatric Research 1990;28(6):631-640.

46. Butte NF, Wong, WW, Garza C et al: Energy Requirements of Breastfed Infants. Journal of the American College of Nutrition 1991;10(3):190-195.

47. Cable TA, Rothenberger LA: Breastfeeding behavioral patterns among La Leche League mothers: A descriptive survey. Pediatrics 1984;73(6):830-835.

48. Calvo EB, Galindo AC, Aspres NB: Iron status in exclusively breastfed infants. Pediatrics 1992;90(3):375-379.

49. Cant AJ: Diet and the prevention of childhood allergic disorders. J Human Nutri: Applied Nutri 1984;38(A):455-468.

50. Cant AJ, Bailes JA, Marsden RA: Cow's milk, soya milk, and goat's milk in a mother's diet causing eczema and diarrhea in her breastfed infant. Acta Paediatr Scand 1985;74:467-468.

51. Cant AJ, Marsden RA, Kilshaw PJ: Egg and cow's milk hypersensitivity in exclusively breastfed infants with eczema, and detection of egg protein in breast milk. Brit Med J 1985;291:932-935.

52. Cashore WJ, Stern L: The management of hyperbilirubinemia. Clin Perinato 1984;11: 339-357.

53. Chaney NE, Franke J, Wadlington WB: Cocaine convulsions in a breastfeeding baby. J Pediatrics 1988;112(1):134-135.

54. Chapman JJ, Macey MJ, Keegan M et al: Concerns of breastfeeding mothers from birth to four months. Nurs Research 1985; 34(6):374-377.

55. Chasnoff IJ, Lewis DE, Squires L: Cocaine intoxication in a breastfed infant. Pediatrics 1987;80(6)836-838.

56. Chilvers CED: Breastfeeding and risk of breast cancer in young women. BMJ 1993; 307:17-20.

57. Clark LL, Beal VA: Prevalence and duration of breastfeeding in Manitoba. Can Med Assoc J 1982;126:1173-1175.

58. Clemens J, Rao M, Ahmed F et al: Breastfeeding and the risk of life-threatening rotavirus diarrhea: Prevention or postponement? Pediatrics 1993;92(5):680-685.

59. Cole JP: Breastfeeding in the Boston suburbs in relation to personal-social factors. Clin Pediatr 1977;16(4)352-356.

60. Committee on Drugs, American Academy of Pediatrics: The transfer of drugs and other chemicals into human milk. Pediatrics 1994;93(1):137-150.

61. Cooper DW: Antithyroid drugs: To breast-feed or not to breastfeed. Am J Obstet Gynecol 1987;157(2):234-235.

62. Cronenwett L: Nipple Confusion (letter). Pediatrics 1993;92(2):301.

63. Cronenwett L, Stukel T, Kearney M et al: Single daily bottle use in the early weeks postpartum and breastfeeding outcomes. Pediatrics 1992;90(5):760-766.

64. Crowder DS: Maternity nurses' knowledge of factors promoting successful breastfeeding. JOGN Nurs Jan/Feb 1981; 28-30.

65. Cunningham AS, Jelliffe DB, Jelliffe EFP: Breastfeeding and health in the 1980s: A global epidemiologic review. J Pediatr 1991;118(5):659-665.

66. Davis MK, Savitz DA, Graubard BI: Infant feeding and childhood cancer. Lancet 1988;2:365-368.

67. DeCarvalho M, Hall M, Harvey D: Effects of water supplementation on physiological jaundice in breastfed babies. Arch Dis Child 1981;56:568-569.

68. DeCarvalho M, Klaus MH, Merkatz RB: Frequency of breastfeeding and serum bilirubin concentration. Am J Dis Child August 1982;136:737-738.

69. DeCarvalho M, Robertson S, Friedman A, Klaus M: Effect of frequent breastfeeding on early milk production and infant weight gain. Pediatrics 1983;72(3):307-311.

70. Dewey KG, Heinig MJ, Nommsen LA et al: Adequacy of energy intake among breast-fed infants in the DARLING study: Relationships to growth velocity, morbidity, and activity levels. The Journal of Pediatrics 1991;119(4):538-547.

71. Dewey KG, Heinig MJ, Nommsen LA et al: Growth of breastfed and formula fed infants from 0-18 months: The DARLING Study. Pediatrics 1992;89(6):1035-1041.

72. Dewey KG, Heinig MJ, Nommsen LA et al: Zinc status in breastfed infants (letter): Lancet 1992;340:1416-1417.

73. Dilts CL: Nursing management of mastitis due to breastfeeding. JOGN Nurs July/Aug 1985;286-288.

74. Dodgson J: Early identification of potential breastfeeding problems. J Hum Lact 1989;5(2):80-81.

75. Doyl LW, Rickards AL, Kelly EA et al: Breast-feeding and intelligence (letter). Lancet 1992;339:744-745.

76. Duffy LC, Byers TE, Riepenhoff-Talty M et al: The effects of infant feeding on rotavirus-induced gastroenteritis: A prospective study. AJPH 1986;76(3)259-263.

77. Duncan B, Ey J, Holberg CJ et al: Exclusive breastfeeding for at least 4 months protects against otitis media. Pediatrics 1993;91 (5):867-872.

78. Dusdieker LB, Booth BM, Seals BF, Ekwo EE: Investigation of a model for the initiation of breastfeeding in primigravida women. Soc Sci Med 1985;20(7):695-703.

79. Ekbom A, Hsieh C-C, Trichopoulos D et al: Breastfeeding and breast cancer in the offspring. Br J Cancer 1993;67(4):842-845.

80. Ekwo EE, Dusdieker LB, Booth BM: Factors influencing initiation of breastfeeding. Am J Dis Child 1983;137:375-377.

81. Entwisle DR, Doering SG, Reilly TW: Sociopsychological determinants of women's breastfeeding behavior: A replication and extension. Am J Orthopsy 1982;52(2):224-260.

82. Feinstein JM, Berkelhamer JE, Gruszka ME et al: Factors related to early termination of breastfeeding in an urban population. Pediatrics 1986;78(2):210-215.

83. Frank DA, Wirtz SJ, Sorenson JR, Heeren TH: Commercial discharge packs and breastfeeding counseling: Effects on infant feeding practices in a randomized trial. Pediatrics 1987;80(6):845-854.

84. Frantz KB, Fleiss PM, Lawrence RA: Management of the slow-gaining breastfed baby. Resources in Human Nuturing, Monograph No. 1, Denver, CO 1978.

85. Frantz KB, Kalmen BA: Breastfeeding works for cesareans, too. RN 1979;42(12):39-47.

86. Frederick IB: Breastfeeding. Obstet Gyne Annu 1984;13:131-151.

87. Fredrickson D: Nipple Confusion (letter). Pediatrics 1993;92(2):300-301.

88. Friel J, Hudson N: The effect of a promotion campaign on attitudes of adolescent females towards breastfeeding. Can J Pub Hlth 1989:80(3):195-199.

89. Gale R, Dollberg S: Breastfeeding of term infants three-hour vs four-hour non-demand: A randomized controlled reappraisal of hospital based feeding schedules. Clin Pediatr 1989;28(10):458-460.

90. Gambon RC, Lentze MJ, Rossi E: Megaloblastic anaemia in one of monozygous twins breastfed by their vegetarian mother. Eur J Pediatr 1986;145:570-571.

91. Gerrard JW, Shenassa M: Food allergy: Two common types as seen in breast and formula fed babies. Annals of Allergy 1983; 50:375-379.

92. Ghaeli P, Kaufman MB: Oral antihistamines/decongestants and breastfeeding. J Hum Lact 1993;9(4):261-2.

93. Gielsen AC, Faden RR, O'Campo P et al: Maternal employment during the early post-partum period: Effects on initiation and continuation of breastfeeding. Pediatrics 1991;87(3):298-305.

94. Goldberg RJ, Cutie AJ: Your CE topic this month (no. 6) drug excretion into human milk: Part 1. J Pract Nurs 1983;33:24-31.

95. Goldfarb J, Tibbetts E: Breastfeeding handbook. Enslow Publishers, Hillside, NJ 1980.

96. Grossman L, Larsen, Alexander J: Breastfeeding among low income high-risk women. Clin Pediatr 1989;28(1):38-42.

97. Grumach AS, Carmona RC, Lazarotti D et al: Immunological factors in milk from Brazilian mothers delivering small-for-date term neonates. Acta Paediatr 1993;82:284-290.

98. Gulick EE: Infant health and breastfeeding. Pediatric Nursing 1983;9(5):359-389.

99. Habicht JP, DaVanzo J, Butz WP: Mother's milk and sewage: Their interactive effects on infant mortality. Pediatrics 1988;81 (3):456-461.

100. Hahn-Zoric M, Fulconis F, Minoli I et al: Antibody responses to parenteral and oral vaccines are impaired by conventional and low protein formulas as compared to breastfeeding. Acta Paediatr Scand 1990; 79:1137-1142.

101. Hall JM: Influencing breastfeeding success. JOGN Nurs 1978;28-32.

102. Harsten G, Prellner K: Recurrent otitis media: A prospective study of children during the first three years of life. Acta Otolaryngologica Stockh 1989;107(1-2):111-119.

103. Hawkins LM, Nichols FH, Tanner JL: Predictors of the duration of breastfeeding in low-income women. Birth 1987;14(4):209.

104. Heery LB: Nipple Confusion (letter). Pediatrics 1993;92(2): 299.

105. Heinig MJ, Nommsen LA, Peerson JM et al: Energy and protein intakes of breastfed and formula fed infants during the first year of life and their association with growth velocity: The DARLING Study. Am J Clin Nutr 1993;58:152-161.

106. Hendershot E: Trends in breastfeeding. Pediatrics 1984;74(4 Pt 2):591-602.

107. Hewat RJ, Ellis DJ: Breastfeeding as maternal-child team effort: Women's perceptions. Hlth Care Women Intl 1984;5:437-452.

108. Hide DW, Guyer BM: Clinical manifestations of allergy related to breast- and cow's milk- feeding. Pediatrics 1985;76(6):973-974.

109. Hill PD, Aldag JC: Insufficient milk supply among black and white breastfeeding mothers. Research in Nursing and Hlth 1993;16:203-211

110. Hillervik-Lindquist C, Hofvander Y, Sjolin S: Studies on perceived breast milk insufficiency: Consequences for breast milk consumption and growth. Acta Paediatr Scand 1991;80:297-303.

111. Hills-Bonczyk SG, Avery MD, Savik K et al: Women's experiences with combining breastfeeding and employment. Journal of Nurse-Midwifery 1993;38(5):257-266.

112. Holmes GE, Hassanein KM, Miller HC: Factors associated with infections among breastfed babies and babies fed proprietary milks. Pediatrics 1983;72(3):300-306.

113. Hoppu K, Neuvonen PJ, Korte T: Disopyramide and breastfeeding (letter). Br J Clin Pharmacol 1986;21(5):553.

114. Host A, Husby S: A prospective study of cow's milk allergy in exclusively breastfed infants: Incidence pathogenetic role of early inadvertent exposure to cow's milk formula, and characteristics of bovine milk protein in human milk. Acta Pediatr Scand 1988; 77(5):663-670.

115. Houston MJ: Breastfeeding: Success or failure. J Adv Nurs 1981;6:447-457.

116. Houston M, Field P: Practices and policies in the initiation of breastfeeding. J Obstet Gynecol Neonatal Nurs 1988;17(6):418-424.

117. Houston MJ, Howie PW: Home support for the breastfeeding mother. J Hlth Visitor 1981;54(6):378.

118. Houston MJ, Howie PW, McNeilly AS: Factors affecting the duration of breastfeeding: 1. Measurement of breast milk intake in the first week of life. Early Hum Dev 1983;8:49-54.

119. Houston MJ, Howie PW, Smart L et al: Factors affecting the duration of breastfeeding: 2. Early feeding practices and social class. Early Hum Dev 1983;8:55-63.

120. Howie PW: Breastfeeding: A natural method for child spacing. Am J Obstet Gynecol 1991;165:1990-1991.

121. Ito S, Blajchman A, Stephenson M et al: Prospective follow-up of adverse reactions in breastfed infants exposed to maternal medication. Am J Obstet Gynecol 1993; 168(5):1393-1399.

122. Jacobson SW, Jacobson JL: Breastfeeding and intelligence (letter). Lancet 1992; 339:926.

123. Jakaabsson I, Lindberg T: Cow's milk proteins cause infantile colic in breastfed infants: A double-blind crossover study. Pediatrics 1983;71(2):268-271.

124. Jelliffe DB: Recent developments in breastfeeding. Med J Malaysia 1986;41 (1):59-63.

125. Jelliffe DB, Jelliffe EFP: "Breast is best": Modern meanings. N Engl J Med 1977; 297:912-915.

126. Jelliffe DB, Jelliffe EFP: Human milk in the modern world. Oxford University Press, Oxford, England 1978.

127. Jelliffe DB, Jelliffe EFP: Recent scientific knowledge concerning breastfeeding. Rev Epidem et Sante Publ 1983;31:367-373.

128. Jelliffe EFP: Programmes to promote breastfeeding. Med J Malaysia 1986;41 (1):64-71.

129. John AM, Martorell R: Incidence and duration of breastfeeding in Mexican/American infants. Am J Clin Nutr 1989;50(4):868-874.

130. Jones AW: Alcohol in mother's milk (letter). N Engl J Med 1992;326(11):766.

131. Jones D: Breastfeeding problems. Nurs Times Aug 1974;53-54.

132. Jones DA: Attitudes of breastfeeding mothers: A survey of 649 mothers. Soc Sci Med 1986;23(11):1151-1156.

133. Jordan PL: Breastfeeding as a risk factor for fathers. JOGN Nurs March/April 1986;94-97.

134. Karjalainen J, Martin J, Knip M et al: A bovine albumin peptide as a possible trigger of insulin-dependent diabetes mellitus. N Enl J Med 1992;327:302-307.

135. Karra MV, Auerbach KG, Olson L et al: Hospital infant feeding practices in metropolitan Chicago: An evaluation of five of the "Ten Steps to Successful Breastfeeding". J Am Diet Assoc 1993;93 (12):1437-1439.

136. Kaufman K, Hall L: Influences of the social network on choice and duration of breastfeeding in mothers of pre-term infants. Res Nurs Hlth 1989;12(3):149-159.

137. Kaufman R, Foxman B: Mastitis among lactating women: Occurrence and risk factors. Soc Sci Med 1991;33(6):701-705.

138. Kearney M: Identifying psychosocial obstacles to breastfeeding success. J Obstet Gynecol Neonatal Nurs 1988;17(2):98-105.

139. Kelly M: Will mothers breastfeed longer if health visitors give them more support? Hlth Visit 1983;56:407-409.

140. Kemper K, Forsyth B, McCarty P: Jaundice, terminating breastfeeding and the vulnerable child. Pediatrics 1989;84(5):773-778.

141. Kennedy K, Rivera R: Consensus statement on the use of breastfeeding as a family planning method. Contraception 1989;39(5):477-495.

142. Kennedy KI, Parenteau-Carreau S, Flynn A et al: The natural family planning-lactational amenorrhea method interface: Observations from a prospective study of breastfeeding users of family planning. Am J Obstet Gynecol 1991;165:2020-2026.

143. Kennedy KI, Visness CM: Contraceptive efficacy of lactational amenorrhea. Lancet 1992;339:227-230.

144. Kirksey A, Groziak SM: Maternal drug use: Evaluation of risks to breastfed infants. World Rev Nutr Diet 1984;43:60-79.

145. Kivlahan C, James EJP: The natural history of neonatal jaundice. Pediatrics 1984; 74(3):364-370.

146. Kovar MG, Serdula MK et al: Review of the epidemiologic evidence for an association between infant feeding and infant health. Pediatrics 1984;74(4 Pt 2):615-638.

147. Krugman S: Viral hepatitis: 1985 update. Pediatrics in Review 1985;7(1):3-11.

148. Kurini N, Shiono PH: Does maternal employment affect breastfeeding? Am J Public Hlth 1989;79(9):1247-1250.

149. Kurini N, Shiono PH: Early formula supplementation of breastfeeding. Pediatrics 1991;88(4):745-750.

150. Kurini N, Shiono PH, Rhoads GG: Breastfeeding incidence and duration in black and white women. Pediatrics 1988; 81(3)365-371.

151. La Leche League International: The womanly art of breastfeeding. La Leche League International, Franklin Park, IL 1981.

152. Labbok M, Simon S: A community study of a decade of in-hospital breastfeeding promotion. Am J Prev Med 1988;4(2):62-67.

153. Labbok MH, Stallings RY, Shah F et al: Ovulation method use during breastfeeding: Is there increased risk of unplanned pregnancy? Am J Obstet Gynecol 1991; 165:2031-2036.

154. Lascari AD: "Early" breastfeeding jaundice: Clinical significance. J Pediatr 1986; 108:156-158.

155. Lawrence RA: Breastfeeding: A guide for the medical profession. Mosby-Year Book, Inc., St. Louis MO. 4th Edition 1994.

156. Lawrence RA: Breastfeeding: A guide for the medical profession. The C.V. Mosby Company, St. Louis, MO 1985.

157. Lawrence RA: Breastfeeding trends: A cause for action (letter). Pediatrics 1991; 88(4):867-868.

158. Lawrence RA: Practices and attitudes toward breastfeeding among medical professionals. Pediatrics 1982;70:912-920.

159. Layde F, Webster L: The independent associations of parity, age of first full-term pregnancy and duration of breastfeeding with the risk of breast cancer. J Clin Epidemiol 1989;42(10):963-975.

160. L'Esperance C, Frantz K: Time limitations for early breastfeeding. JOGN Nurs 1985; March/April:114-118.

161. Lee KS, Gartner LM: Management of unconjugated hyperbilirubinemia in the newborn. Semin Liver Dis 1983;3:52-64.

162. Leibhaber M, Lewiston NJ, Asquith MT, Sunshine P: Comparison of bacterial contamination with two methods of human milk collection. J Pediatrics 1978;92(2):237.

163. Lethbridge DJ: The use of breastfeeding as a contraceptive. J Obstet Gynecol Neonatal Nurs 1989;18(1):31-37.

164. Lifschitz CH, Hawkins HK, Guerra C, Byrd N: Anaphylactic shock due to cow's milk protein hypersensitivity in a breastfed infant. J Ped Gastro Nutr 1988;7:141-144.

165. Little R, Anderson K: Maternal alcohol use during breastfeeding and infant mental and motor development at one year. N Eng J Med 1989;321(17):425-430.

166. Lodinova-Zadnikova R, Slavikova M, Tlaskalova-Hogenova H et al: The antibody response in breastfed and non-breastfed infants after artificial colonization of the intestine with escherichia coli 083. Pediatric Res 1991;29(4):396-399.

167. Lucas A, Morley R, Cole TJ et al: Breast milk and subsequent intelligence quotient in children born preterm. Lancet 1991; 339:261-264.

168. Mackey S, Fried PA: Infant breast and bottle feeding practices: some related factors and attitudes. Can J Pub Hlth 1981;72:312-318.

169. MacLaughlin S, Strelnick EG: Breastfeeding and working outside the home. Issues Compr Pediatr Nurs 1984;7:67-81.

170. Maisels MJ, Gifford K: Neonatal jaundice in full-term infants: Role of breastfeeding and other causes. Am J Dis Child 1983;137:561-562.

171. Maisels MJ, Gifford K: Normal serum bilirubin levels in the newborn and the effect of breastfeeding. Pediatrics 1986;78(5):837-843.

172. Maisels MJ, Gifford K, Antle CE, Leib GR: Jaundice in the healthy newborn infant: A new approach to an old problem. Pediatrics 1988;81(4):505-511.

173. Maisels MJ, Vain N, Acquavita AM et al: The effect of breastfeeding frequency on serum bilirubin levels. Am J Obstet Gynecol 1994; 170(3):880-883.

174. Marild S, Jodal U, Hanson L: Breastfeeding and urinary-tract infection (letter). Lancet 1990;336(8720):942.

175. Marmet C, Shell E: Training neonates to suck correctly. MCN 1984;9:401-407.

176. Martinez GA, Dodd, DA: 1981 milk feeding patterns in the United States during the first 12 months of life. Pediatrics 1983;71(2):166-170.

177. Martinez GA, Krieger FW: 1984 milk feeding patterns in the United States. Pediatrics 1985;76:1004-1008.

178. Martinez GA, Nelezienski JP: 1980 Update: The recent trend in breastfeeding. Pediatrics 1981;67(2):260-263.

179. Martinez GA, Stahle DA: The recent trend in milk feeding among WIC infants. AJPH 1982;72(1):68-71.

180. Martinez JC, Maisels MJ, Otheguy L et al: Hyperbilirubinemia in the breastfed newborn: A controlled trial of four interventions. Pediatrics 1993;91(2):470-473.

181. McKenna R, Cole ER, Vasan U: Is warfarin sodium contraindicated in the lactating mother? Pediatrics 1983;103(2):325-327.

182. Mennella J, Beauchamp G: Effects of beer on breastfed infants. JAMA 1993; 269(13):1637.

183. Michaelse KF, Larsen PS, Thomsen BL et al: The Copenhagen Cohort Study on Infant Nutrition and Growth: Breast milk intake, human milk macronutrient content, and influencing factors. Am J Clin Nutr 1994;59:600-611.

184. Miller SA, Chopra JG: Problems with human milk and infant formulas. Pediatrics 1984;74(4 Pt 2):639-648.

185. Minchin M: Positioning for breastfeeding. Birth 1989;16(2):67-73.

186. Morgan J: A study of mothers' breastfeeding concerns. Birth 1986;13(2):104-108.

187. Morrow-Tlucak M, Haude R: Breastfeeding and cognitive development in the first two years of life. Soc Sci Med 1988;26(6):635-639.

188. Morse J, Bottorff J: Patterns of breastfeeding and work: The Canadian experience. Can J Pub Hlth 1989;80(3):182-188.

189. Mulford C: Infant feeding and infectious disease (letter). Pediatrics 1990;86(5):806-807.

190. Mulford C: Nipple confusion (letter). Pediatrics 1993;92(2):298-299.

191. Myers MG, Foman SJ, Koontz FP et al: Respiratory and gastrointestinal illnesses in breast- and formula-fed infants. Am J Dis Child 1984;138:629-632.

192. National Survey of Family Growth: Trends in breastfeeding among American mothers. U.S. Dept. of Health, Education and Welfare Pub No. (PHS)79-1979:1979.

193. Neifert M, Gray J: Effects of two types of hospital feeding gift packs on duration of breastfeeding among adolescent mothers. J Adolesc Hlth Care 1988;9(5):411-413.

194. Neifert MR, Gray J: Factors influencing breastfeeding among adolescents. J Adolesc Hlth Care 1988;9(6):470-473.

195. Neifert MR, McDonough SL, Neville MC: Failure of lactogenesis associated with placental retention. Am J Obstet Gynecol 1981;140:477-478.

196. Neifert MR, Seacat JM: A guide to successful breastfeeding. Contemporary Pediatrics 1986;3(7):26-45.

197. Neifert MR, Seacat JM: Medical management of successful breastfeeding. Pediatr Clin North Am 1986;33:743-762.

198. Neifert MR, Seacat JM, Jobe WE: Lactation failure due to insufficient glandular development of the breast. Pediatrics 1985;76(5):823-828.

199. Newcomb PA, Storer BE, Longnecker MP et al: Lactation and a reduced risk of premenopausal breast cancer. N Eng J Med 1994;330(2):81-87.

200. Newman J: Nipple confusion (letter). Pediatrics 1993;92(2):297-298.

201. Nutrition During Lactation, Institute of Medicine report: National Academy of Sciences, Committee on Nutritional Status During Pregnancy and Lactation, Food and Nutrition Board, National Academy Press, 1991.

202. Ojofeitmi EO: The effect of early initiation of colostrum feeding on proliferation of intestinal bacteria in neonates. Clin Ped 1982;21(1):39.

203. Osborn LM, Bolus R: Breastfeeding and jaundice in the first week of life. J Fam Prac 1985;20(5):475-480.

204. Oski FA: Iron deficiency, facts and fallacies. Pediatr Clin North Am 1985;32:493-497.

205. Perez-Escamilla R, Pollitt E, Lonnerdal B et al: Infant feeding policies in maternity wards and their effect on breastfeeding success: An analytical overview. Am J Public Hlth 1994;84(1):89-97.

206. Peters DC, Worthington-Roberts: Infant feeding practices in middle-class breast-feeding and formula feeding mothers. Birth 1982;9(2):91-95.

207. Petschek MA, Barber-Madden R: Promoting prenatal care and breastfeeding in the workplace. Occup Hlth Nurs 1985;33:86-89.

208. Pisacane A, Graziano L, Zona G: Breastfeeding and urinary tract infection (letter). Lancet 1990;336(8706):50.

209. Pisacane A, Liberatore G, Mazzareool G et al: Breastfeeding and urinary tract infection. The Journal of Pediatrics 1992;120 (1):87-89.

210. Pittard WB, Anderson DM, Cerutti ER: Bacteriostatiz qualities of human milk. The Journal of Pediatrics 1985;107:240-243.

211. Pizarro F, Yip R, Dallman PR et al: Iron status with different infant feeding regimens: Relevance to screening and prevention of iron deficiency. The Journal of Pediatrics 1991;118(5):687-692.

212. Platzker ACD, Lew CD, Stewart D: Drug administration via breast milk. Hosp Prac Sept 1980;111-121.

213. Popkins BM, Adair L, Akin JS et al: Breastfeeding and diarrheal morbidity. Pediatrics 1990;86(6):874-882.

214. Pratt HF: Breastfeeding and eczema. Early Human Dev 1984;9:283-290.

215. Radius S, Joffe A: Understanding adolescent mothers' feelings about breastfeeding: A study of perceived benefits and barriers. J Adolesc Hlth Care 1988;9(2):156-160.

216. Rassin DK, Richardson J, Baranowski T et al: Incidence of breastfeeding in a low socioeconomic group of mothers in the United States: Ethnic patterns. Pediatrics 1984;73 (2):132-137.

217. Reiff MI, Essoc-Vitale SM: Hospital influences on early infant feeding practices. Pediatrics 1985;76(6):872-878.

218. Reifsnider E, Myers ST: Employed mothers can breastfeed, too! MCN 1985;10:256-259.

219. Reisner SH, Eisenberg NH et al: Maternal medications and breastfeeding. Dev Pharmacol Ther 1983;6:285-304.

220. Reniers JR, Peeters RF, Meheus AZ: Breastfeeding in the industrialized world: Review of the literature. Rev Epidem et Sante Publ 1983;31:375-407.

221. Reves RR: Illnesses in breast- and bottle-fed infants. Am J Dis Child 1986;140:185-186.

222. Riordan J, Auerbach KG, eds: Breastfeeding and human lactation. Jones and Bartlett Publishers, Boston, 1993.

223. Roex AJM, van Loenen AC, Puyenbroek JI, Arts NFT: Secretion of cefoxitin in breast milk following short-term prophylactic administration in caesarean section. Eur J Obstet Gynecol Reprod Biol 1987;25:299-302.

224. Rogan WJ, Gladen BC: Breastfeeding and cognitive development. Early Hum Dev 1993;31:181-193.

225. Romero-Gwyn E, Carias L: Breastfeeding intention and practice among Hispanic mothers in southern California. Pediatrics 1989;84(4):626-632.

226. Rosner AE, Schulman SK: Birth interval among breastfeeding women not using contraceptives. Pediatrics 1990;86(5):747-752

227. Rubin DH, Leventhal JN, Krasilnikoff PA et al: Relationships between infant feeding and infectious illness: A prospective study of infants during the first year of life. Pediatrics 1990;85:464-471.

228. Ryan A, Martinez G: Breastfeeding and the working mother: A profile. Pediatric 1989; 83(4):524-531.

229. Ryan AS, Pratt WF, Wyson JL et al: A comparison of breastfeeding data from the national surveys of family growth and the Ross Laboratories mothers surveys. Am J Public Hlth 1991;81(8):1049-1052.

230. Ryan AS, Rush D, Krieger FW et al: Recent declines in breastfeeding in the United States, 1984 through 1989. Pediatrics 1991;88(4):719-727.

231. Saarinen UM: Prophylaxis for atopic disease: Role of infant feeding. Clin Rev Allergy 1984;2:151-167.

232. Salariya EM, Easton PM, Cater Jl: Duration of breastfeeding after early initiation and frequent feeding. Lancet 1978;1141-1143.

233. Sarett HP, Bain KR, O'Leary JC: Decisions on breastfeeding or formula feeding and trends in infant feeding practices. Am J Dis Child 1983;137:719-725.

234. Schlager TA, Dudley SM, Dunn, ML et al: Breastfeeding and urinary tract infections (letter). The Journal of Pediatrics 1992; 120(2):331.

235. Schlegel AM: Observations on breastfeeding technique: Facts and fallacies. MCN 1983;8:204-208.

236. Schmitt BD: The prevention of sleep problems and colic. Pediatr Clin North Am 1986;33:763-774.

237. Schneider PA: Breast milk jaundice in the newborn. JAMA 1986;255(23):3270-3274.

238. Schulte-Hobein B, Schwartz-Bickenbach D, Abt S et al: Cigarette smoke exposure and development of infants throughout the first year of life: Influence of passive smoking and nursing on cotinine levels in breast milk and infant's urine. Acta Paediatr 1992; 81:550-557.

239. Scott FW: Cow milk and insulin-dependent diabetes mellitus: Is there a relationship? Am J Clin Nutr 1990;51:489-491.

240. Seward J, Serdula MK: Infant feeding and infant growth. Pediatrics 1984;74(4 Pt 2): 728-762.

241. Shiffman M, Seale T: Breast milk composition in women with cystic fibrosis: Report of two cases and a review of the literature. Am J Clin Nutr 1989;49(4):612-617.

242. Sievers E, Oldigs H-D, Dorner K et al: Longitudinal zinc balances in breastfed and formula-fed infants. Acta Paediatr 1992; 81:1-6.

243. Simopoulos AP, Grave GD: Factors associated with the choice and duration of infant feeding practice. Pediatrics 1984;74(4 Pt 2):603-614.

244. Siskind V, Schofield F: Breast cancer and breastfeeding: Results from an Australian case control study. Am J Epidemiol 1989;130(2):229-236.

245. Skeel L, Good M: Mexican cultural beliefs and breastfeeding: A model for assessment and intervention. J Human Lact 1988:4(4):160-163.

246. Smigel K: Breastfeeding linked to decreased cancer risk for mother, child. J Natl Cancer Inst 1988;80(17):1362-1363.

247. Smith JC, Mhango CG, Warren CW et al: Trends in the incidence of breastfeeding for Hispanics of Mexican origin and Anglos on the US/Mexico border. AJPH 1982;72(1):59-61.

248. Snider DE, Powell KE: Should women taking antituberculosis drugs breastfeed? Arch Intern Med 1984;144:589-590.

249. Stahl MD, Guida DA: Slow weight gain in the breastfed infant: Management options. Pediatr Nurs 1984;10:117-121.

250. Stahlberg MR: Breastfeeding and social factors. Acta Paediatr Scand 1985;74:36-39.

251. Storr G: Prevention of nipple tenderness and breast engorgement in the postpartum period. J Obstet Gynecol Neonatal Nurs 1988;17(3):203-209.

252. Tainio V, Savilahti E: Risk factors for infantile recurrent otitis media: Atopy but not type of feeding. Pediatr Res 1988;23(5):509-512.

253. Tamminen T, Verronen P, Saarikoski S et al: The influence of perinatal factors on breastfeeding. Acta Paediatr Scand 1983;72:9-12.

254. The Early Feeds: Human milk vs. formula and bovine milk. Summary of workshop on current issues in feeding the normal infant. Pediatrics 1985;(suppl):157-159.

255. Thomsen AC, Espersen T, Maigaard S: Course and treatment of milk stasis, noninfectious inflammation of the breast, and infectious mastitis in nursing women. Am J Obstet Gynecol 1984;149:492-495.

256. Tully J, Dewey KG: Private fears, global loss: A cross-cultural study of the insufficient milk syndrome. Med Anthro 1985; Summer:225-243.

257. Tupasi T, Velmonte M: Determinants of morbidity and mortality due to respiratory infections: Implications for intervention. J Infect Dis 1988;157(4):615-623.

258. van den Bogaard C, van den Hoogen HJM, Huygen FJA et al: The relationship between breastfeeding and early childhood morbidity in a general population. Fam Med 1991; 23:510-515.

259. Victora CG, Tomasi E, Olinto MTA et al: Use of pacifiers and breastfeeding duration. Lancet 1993;341:404-6.

260. Victoria C, Smith P: Infant feeding and deaths due to diarrhea: A case control study. Am J Epidemiol 1989;129(5):1032-1041.

261. Walker M: Management of selected early breastfeeding problems seen in clinical practice. Birth 1989;16(3):148-158.

262. Walker M: Nipple confusion (letter). Pediatrics 1993;92(2):297.

263. Walker WA: Absorption of protein and protein fragments in the developing intestine: Role in immunologic/allergic reactions. Pediatrics 1985;75(suppl):167-171.

264. Walravens PA, Chakar A, Mokni R et al: Zinc supplements in breastfed infants. Lancet 1992;340(8821):683-685.

265. Weinberg RJ, Tipton G, Klish WJ, Brown MR: Effect of breastfeeding on morbidity in rotavirus gastroenteritis. Pediatrics 1984; 74(2):250-253.

266. Welch MJ, Phelps DL, Osher AB: Breastfeeding by a mother with cystic fibrosis. Pediatrics 1981;67(5):664.

267. West CP: Factors influencing the duration of breastfeeding. J Biol Sci 1980;12:325-331.

268. Whitfield M: Validity of routine clinical test weighing. Arch Dis Child 1981;56:91.

269. Wiberg B, Humble K: Long-term effect on mother-infant behavior of extra contract during the first hour postpartum. Scand J Soc Med 1989;17(2):181-191.

270. Widstrom A-M, Thingstrom-Paulsson J: The position of the tongue during rooting reflexes elicited in newborn infants before the first suckle. Acta Paediatr 1993;82:281-283.

271. Wilson N, Hamburger R: Allergy to cow's milk in the first year of life and its prevention. Ann Allergy 1988;61(5):323-327.

272. Winikoff B, Laukaran VH, Myers D, Stone R: Dynamics of infant feeding: Mothers, professionals, and the institutional context in a large urban hospital. Pediatrics 1986; 77(3):357-365.

273. Woolridge M, Fisher C: Colic, "overfeeding" and symptoms of lactose malabsorption in the breastfed baby: A possible artifact of feed management. Lancet 1988;2 (8607):382-384.

274. Worthington-Roberts BS, Vermeersch J, Williams SR: Nutrition in pregnancy and lactation. Times Mirror/Mosby College Publishing, St. Louis, MO 1985.

275. Wright A, Holbert C: Infant feeding practices among middle class Anglos and Hispanics. Pediatrics 1988;82(3):496-503.

276. Wright HJ, Walker PC: Prediction of duration of breastfeeding in primiparas. J Epidemiol Comm Hlth 1983;37:89-94.

277. Yeung DL, Pennell MD, Leung M, Hall J: Breastfeeding: Prevalence and influencing factors. Can J Pub Hlth 1981;72:323-330.

278. Yoo K, Tajima K, Hiros K et al: Independent protective effect of lactation against breast cancer: A case-control study in Japan. Am J Epidemiol 1992;135:726-733.

— OTHER CENTER INDEX PUBLICATIONS —

REPRODUCTIVE HEALTH

Managing Contraceptive Pill Patients - 8th ed. – Dickey
Contraceptive Surgery for Men and Women - 2nd ed. – Moss/AVSC
Endometriosis: *The Enigmatic Disease* — Corson
Estrogen Replacement Therapy User Guide — Gambrell
Family Planning at Your Fingertips — Hatcher, et al
Gynecological Care Manual for HIV Positive Women — Denenberg
Management of Infertility: *A Clinician's Manual* - 2nd ed. – Cohen
Menopause: Clinical Concepts - 2nd ed. - London & Chihal
Managing Danazol Patients - 2nd ed. — Dickey
Hormone Replacement Therapy - 4th ed. — Gambrell
Oral Contraceptive User Guide - 2nd ed. – Dickey
Safe Sex: *A Guide to Condoms* - 2nd ed. – Brackett

CARDIOLOGY

Cholesterol Treatment: *User Guide to Lipid Disorder Management* - 2nd ed. — Leaf
Emergency Cardiac Maneuvers - 2nd ed. — Bartecchi
Hypertension Treatment User Guide - 2nd ed. — Kaplan
Management of Heart Failure — Cohn & Kubo
Management of Hypertension - 6th ed. — Kaplan

GENERAL MEDICINE

A Manual on Drug Dependence — Nahas
A Practical Anesthesia Information Guide — Jerome
Arthritis Therapy: *A Clinician's Manual* — Kantor
Assessment and Management of the Suicidal Adolescent - Clayton
Breast Disease in Women and Men — Shuler
Handbook of Headache Disorders - 2nd ed. — Elkind
Management of Aneurysmal Subarachnoid Hemorrhage — Fosset
Management of Diabetes Mellitus - 3rd ed. — Schwartz & Schwartz
Mid-Life Sexuality: *Enrichment and Problem Solving* — Semmens
Projective Psychodiagnostic Assessment — Caldwell & Dixon
Primary Mental Health Care — Behrman✱

EDUCATION

Accelerated Learning: *How You Learn Determines What You Learn* — Swartz
Chief Executive Officer's Guide for Health Facility Development - 2nd ed. — Weeks
Children with Special Needs - 2nd ed. — Bradway & Block
Infection Prevention for Family Planning Service Programs — Tietjen, Cronin & McIntosh (JHPIEGO) ✱
Resilience Enhancement for the Resident Physician — Messner✱
Travel Well: *a gourmet guide to healthy travel* — Kaplan ✱

✱Not Center-Indexed Publications